integrative medicine for

ALZHEIMER'S

The breakthrough
natural treatment plan
that prevents Alzheimer's
using nutritional Lithium

James Greenblatt, MD

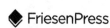 FriesenPress

Suite 300 - 990 Fort St
Victoria, BC, V8V 3K2
Canada

www.friesenpress.com

ISBN
978-1-5255-3997-8 (Hardcover)
978-1-5255-3998-5 (Paperback)
978-1-5255-3999-2 (eBook)

1. Medical, Psychiatry, Psychopharmacology

Distributed to the trade by The Ingram Book Company

DISCLAIMER

The information presented in this book has not been evaluated or approved by the U.S. Food and Drug Administration. The products discussed in this book are not intended to diagnose, treat, cure, or prevent any disease.

The information reviewed in this book is designed to provide information on currently available research on low-dose lithium. This book is not intended, nor should it be used, as a substitute for the medical advice of physicians. The reader should regularly consult a physician in matters relating to his/her health and particularly with respect to any symptoms that may require diagnosis or medical attention. Nutritional supplements should be taken under the supervision of a health care professional.

DEDICATION

This book is dedicated to the scientists and clinicians that have challenged the pharmaceutical treatment models of Alzheimer's and have begun to understand that prevention is possible.

"Lithium has literally been everywhere forever ...."
—Eric Jakobsson

TABLE OF CONTENTS

INTRODUCTION

We are living in exciting times. In the midst of a scientific revolution in understanding brain health, the research that has fueled dramatic developments in neuroscience is finally influencing the clinical practice of medicine. Physicians and the public now have much greater understanding than ever before of the intricate processes that keep the brain healthy as well as those that undermine it. Our new knowledge from the field of neuroscience provides hope for treating diseases that have until now seemed hopeless. One of these is Alzheimer's disease.

These are also exciting times to be a psychiatrist. In medical school and fellowship training in psychiatry, we learned to diagnose conditions based on general symptoms, with little awareness of biochemical individuality or underlying biological mechanisms that might contribute to the development of certain symptoms. During that period, treatment decisions did not consider genetics, metabolism, or nutrition as risk factors worth intervening.

Fortunately, implications of new knowledge about the brain are shifting medical culture. Neuroscience research is illuminating the contribution of nutrition to brain health and function. Mapping the genetic code opens a window of knowledge about hereditary predispositions to diseases and even to the ability to influence those genetic tendencies. Today, we have the tools to understand the patient's individual biochemistry and its interplay with diseases that affect the brain.

My psychiatric practice is based on integrative medicine, which relies on insights from current scientific research combined with natural strategies. Integrative medicine is a therapeutic approach to healing that treats the whole patient as an individual. It differs from conventional medicine, which tends to view and treat each body system as an isolated entity and—in the case of psychiatry—the mind as separate from the body.

While integrative medicine leverages important tools that many physicians wouldn't think of because they are outside the confines of the traditional discipline, it is solidly based in scientific medicine. It, more thoroughly than conventional treatment, aims to assess all factors that may contribute to a problem.

One aspect of integrative medicine is nutritional psychiatry, founded on the conviction that identifying and correcting nutritional deficiencies will restore optimal function of the body and brain. I now incorporate nutritional interventions into my psychiatric work with patients. Nutritional medication has historically been considered "alternative" medicine. Holding on to this outdated view, psychiatrists continued to lag behind the rest of medicine in incorporating nutritional interventions and therapies into treatment. The last decade and a half of scientific research have decisively established that nutritional medicine should no longer be labelled "alternative."

> No longer relegated to the arena of "alternative medicine," nutritional psychiatry has emerged as a powerful and scientifically backed medical discipline able to assess the entirety of mental health phenomena.

We now know that nutrients support the biochemical reactions necessary for optimal brain function. We know this from an exponentially increasing number of research studies, and I know this from my day-to-day clinical experience. The improvement I witness as my patients get better affirms the encouraging

> There is light on the horizon when it comes to dementia and Alzheimer's research, nutritional interventions capable of turning the tide on these devastating, debilitating conditions. The most exciting of these is lithium.

results of recent research. Nutritional psychiatry is *integrative* to the extent that we weave this insight into our existing web of medical knowledge.

I have written books on nutrition and anorexia, binge eating, depression, and attention deficit hyperactivity disorder—familiar psychiatric subjects and diagnoses. Alzheimer's disease, on the other hand, may seem an unusual subject for a psychiatrist to tackle. Psychiatry is not often the first avenue explored for treatment. I am writing this book because in my work with patients with mood disorders, I have become aware of the tremendous power of nutritional interventions for dementia and Alzheimer's disease. The most important of these is the simple, brain-protecting nutrient lithium.

Though not the usual province of a psychiatrist, Alzheimer's disease concerns me as a physician, a family member, a taxpayer, and—along with the rest of the population—someone who is aging. With limited treatment options available, it is worth making the research more widely available to those who can benefit from it.

You may have picked up this book because you have a personal association with Alzheimer's disease as well. Maybe you have a parent or grandparent whose once clear thinking seems to have receded behind a fog, out of reach. Maybe you are a caretaker whose time and life are overwhelmed by the needs of an increasingly disabled family member with dementia. Or maybe you are rather worried about your own tendency to misplace the car keys.

As a physician, I have strong respect for scientific evidence. In the chapters that follow, I base all observations and recommendations on the results of scientific research. I urge you to use solid peer-reviewed research as your standard for accepting and following any prevention and treatment suggestions you hear or read about. Especially with an almost universally dreaded disease like Alzheimer's, many Internet marketers offer extravagant promises of cure. Unfortunately, wishing they were true doesn't make it so.

But there is realistic good news about Alzheimer's disease. I am excited to tell you about recent promising research showing lithium's abilities to protect the brain from the deterioration that impairs cognition and speeds up memory loss. I will also tell you about sound research studies of other nutritional supplements that can fortify the health of your brain. I'll discuss tests you can take to discover genetic mutations and vitamin and mineral deficiencies that can damage brain cells. Finally, we'll look at lifestyle choices that enhance brain health from a psychiatric perspective.

You will see that there is hope for protecting yourself from Alzheimer's disease. But first let's look at why this protection is so important.

PART 1
UNDERSTANDING
ALZHEIMER'S DISEASE

1
THE BURDEN OF ALZHEIMER'S

One writer compared it to walking into the middle of a movie: the theater is dark, and people are laughing at something you don't understand because you don't know what has happened or where things are going. This brief moment of disorientation for the late-arriving movie-goer is what life itself is like for people with Alzheimer's disease. No wonder people with Alzheimer's often become paranoid and withdraw. How terrifying it must be to retreat into the citadel of the self only to find it crumbling from within.

The trajectory of Alzheimer's disease is grim. As of this writing, a diagnosis of Alzheimer's leads down a certain path to cognitive decline and, eventually, to death. A once vital individual disappears into the darkness. To sense the magnitude of this burden, multiply this loss millions of times.

> A diagnosis of Alzheimer's leads down a certain path to cognitive decline and, eventually, to death. As relentless and burdensome as this disease truly is, it can be effectively delayed by the humble mineral lithium.

The human brain, with its impressive capacity to create, imagine, and solve complex problems, also has a physiological tendency towards deterioration. Our longer life span and larger brain size come with an evolutionary price: as far as researchers can tell, humans are the only animals vulnerable to neurodegenerative brain disorders such as Alzheimer's disease.

The prevalence of Alzheimer's disease is increasing at an alarming rate. In 2012, the disease affected 35.6 million people worldwide.[1] The World Health Organization predicts that the number of people with Alzheimer's will double every 20 years, to 65.7 million by 2030 and 115.4 million by 2050.[1] Every four seconds, another patient in the world is diagnosed with Alzheimer's.[1]

In 2018, about 5.7 million Americans, 5.5 million of them aged 65 and older, are living with dementia.[2] This means that one in 10 people, or 10% of people 65 and older, have Alzheimer's disease. Almost two-thirds of Americans with Alzheimer's are women,[2] and African-Americans are about twice as likely to have Alzheimer's or other forms of dementia as older whites.[3]

In the United States, Alzheimer's disease is the sixth leading cause of death.[4] It is the only cause of death in the top 10 that cannot be prevented, cured, or even slowed by pharmaceutical intervention.[4] Contrary to common public understanding, it does not strike elderly people exclusively; of all Americans living with Alzheimer's dementia in 2018, at least 200,000 are younger than 65.[5]

The burden of Alzheimer's disease takes a toll well beyond the life of the individual with the diagnosis. Perhaps no other disease exacts a greater toll from loved ones. Whereas most diseases—even terminal ones—leave the individual in command of decisions affecting their care, one of the particular difficulties of Alzheimer's is that others must take the responsibility for decisions—sometimes under great protest from the person with the disease.

The escalating care demands for a person with Alzheimer's led Sherwin Nuland, writing in *How We Die,* to call this disease a scourge that seems specifically designed to test the human spirit.[6] Family caregivers can be "sidetracked from the broad sunlit avenues of ongoing life, remaining trapped for years, each in its own excruciating cul de sac," he wrote.[6] Last year in the United States, friends and families of people with Alzheimer's disease provided an estimated 18.4 billion hours of unpaid care to their family members or friends with the disease.[7] The annual cost of caring for people with dementia or Alzheimer's is $277 billion.[7] This total could reach $1.1 trillion by the year 2050.[7] In the United States, the costs of caring for people with Alzheimer's disease make up 67% of Medicare and Medicaid total costs.[7]

The burden of Alzheimer's disease is also increasing relative to other diseases. While total death rates fell significantly in the United States from 1980 to 2010, deaths from neurological causes rose significantly.[8] From 2000 to 2010, Alzheimer's disease went from the 25th to the 12th most burdensome disease overall and from 32nd to ninth in terms of years of potential lost life. An estimated 10 million baby boomers—people born between 1946 and 1964—in the United States are expected to have Alzheimer's during their lifetime.[9] An estimated 14 million Americans will live with Alzheimer's by 2025.[7]

> The costs—personal, financial, and societal—of Alzheimer's disease are truly staggering, and the search for cures has implications that extend well beyond the individual with the disease.

Clearly, Alzheimer's and other neurodegenerative disorders have become an urgent international public health issue with disastrous medical, social, and economic consequences.

The Hope of Lithium

Before delving further into the stages and processes of dementia and Alzheimer's, it's important to understand where lithium fits in the puzzle. Even from this place, and perhaps in conjunction with our own personal experiences, we can see the dire consequences of Alzheimer's disease on the individual, family, and public health. Yes, lithium is the same drug used to treat bipolar disorder—but its use here is very different. Lithium is a humble, inexpensive mineral effective in delaying the relentless onslaught of dementia. As is discussed later, a few key points are important to remember. Lithium is a natural element that:

- Supports neurogenesis and increases gray matter
- Enhances cell growth and neuroprotection
- Removes plaques and tangles from cells
- Helps healthy cells survive
- Decreases inflammation
- Is inexpensive and easily accessible

Summary

The trajectory of each individual case of Alzheimer's disease is grim, and the prevalence of the disease is increasing at an alarming rate. Alzheimer's takes a toll beyond the individual patient to family and friends who must care for the patient's increasing needs. In the United States in 2017, the costs of caring for patients with Alzheimer's disease reached $277 billion—or more than a quarter of a trillion dollars. Lithium offers a promising and inexpensive route of prevention, thanks to research into its protective mechanism against neurodegeneration.

Key Points

- Alzheimer's disease now affects 35.6 million people worldwide.
- By 2050, if the current rate of increase continues, 115.4 million people will be living with Alzheimer's disease around the world.
- Family and friends of those who suffer with Alzheimer's in the United States provided 17.9 billion hours of unpaid care last year.
- Alzheimer's disease is a public health crisis with massive medical, social, and economic consequences.
- Lithium is an inexpensive neuroprotective mineral that shows promise as a preventive treatment.

2
ALZHEIMER'S AND DEMENTIA: THE PROGRESSIVE STAGES

Alzheimer's is a *progressive* disease—once it begins, it continues to get worse. (In contrast, a common cold is *not* progressive—once it passes, you return to health.) The symptoms and severity of Alzheimer's disease are measured in stages. While there is not universal consensus on the timing and severity of each stage, there is always an initial stage during which there are no outward symptoms, followed by progressive stages of decline that end in death.

To clarify, the term *dementia* does not define a particular disease but rather a broad range of neurodegenerative symptoms caused by loss of brain cell function. It is characterized by progressive and irreparable shrinking of brain tissue. It starts when cells or neurons designed to work in elaborate collaboration begin to deteriorate and can no longer communicate. Networks of neurons or regions of the brain responsible for specific processes like memory, emotion, or movement become compromised or injured. When certain brain areas no longer function, dementia results.

Core skills impaired in dementia may include:
- Short-term memory
- Judgment and problem solving
- Communication and language
- Ability to focus and pay attention
- Visuospatial perception

Again, there is no consensus about the stages that make up Alzheimer's as a progressive disease. Descriptions vary slightly but are similar in their representation of increasing dementia and associated symptoms. Mayo Clinic, for example, divides Alzheimer's progression along five basic stages.[1]

Stage 1: Preclinical Alzheimer's disease. This initial stage involves no outward signs. Even though symptoms are not yet manifest, imaging techniques can identify beta-amyloid protein deposits. The clustered deposits of beta-amyloid are markers that neuronal damage has occurred. Other specific biomarkers identifiable at this early stage include levels of tau protein in cerebrospinal fluid and brain changes detectable by imaging.

> Alzheimer's may well be the greatest public health scourge of the twenty-first century. The combination of its growing prevalence and its 100% mortality rate makes finding a cure among the most urgent priorities in medicine.

Stage 2: Mild cognitive impairment due to Alzheimer's. People in this stage experience mild changes in thinking ability and may have memory lapses about everyday activities such as conversations, recent events, or appointments. These changes are not yet severe enough to affect work or personal relationships and are difficult to distinguish from the mild cognitive decline associated with normal aging.

Stage 3: Mild dementia due to Alzheimer's. Dementia refers to a wide range of symptoms related to memory loss or other cognitive impairments severe enough to interfere with everyday activities. Often, a person in this stage becomes subdued or withdrawn, particularly in challenging situations. A person without dementia can summon a memory when prompted; a person at this stage of Alzheimer's has great difficulty retrieving a memory, even if prompted.

Stage 4: Moderate dementia due to Alzheimer's. The deterioration of memory and cognitive ability is pronounced and poses a risk to personal safety. The person may not recognize friends and even family members. He or she may wander away from home or grow restless, agitated, or aggressive.

Stage 5: Severe dementia due to Alzheimer's. In this stage, individuals cannot live without constant care. They can no longer speak coherently or understand what is said. They need help with all tasks of daily living. Gradually, the brain loses control over bodily functions. Unless they die from an infection first, Alzheimer's ultimately kills them. Often, families feel that, by the time the patient reaches the last phase, the person they knew has already died. The pain of this protracted phase led writer Linda Combs to call Alzheimer's disease "the long goodbye."[2]

The timeline along which Alzheimer's moves inexorably from mild cognitive impairment to severe dementia varies widely. On average, people live with the disease for eight to 10 years after diagnosis.

> On average, people with Alzheimer's live 8 to 10 years after diagnosis.

Some epidemiologists who study trends predict that Alzheimer's disease will be the greatest public health scourge of the twenty-first century. The combination of its growing prevalence and its 100% mortality rate makes finding a cure among the most urgent priorities in medicine. With vast sums of funding devoted to Alzheimer's research, finding a cure would seem simple: figure out how to prevent plaques and tangles from forming. Unfortunately, the search for a cure has been neither simple nor straightforward.

Summary

Dementia is a broad term used to describe a range of neurodegenerative symptoms caused by brain atrophy. Dementia traits vary depending on the affected location in the brain. Alzheimer's disease is a progressive disease and the most common form of dementia. Because degeneration of brain cells usually occurs first in the hippocampus, the first effects involve memory. As more brain cells atrophy, increasing disorientation is evident. Finally, people with Alzheimer's can no longer connect with the environment, and body systems fail. The disease ends in death.

Key Points

- Alzheimer's disease accounts for 60% to 80% of dementia cases.
- Core skills impaired in dementia include short-term memory, judgment and problem solving, communication and language, focus, and spatial perception.
- Alzheimer's disease develops in a series of predictable stages, from the preclinical phase, when no outward symptoms are present, to mild cognitive impairment; moderate dementia, and severe dementia.
- The timeframe of the disease course varies, with life expectancy after diagnosis of, on average, eight to 10 years.
- The combination of Alzheimer's disease's growing prevalence and its certain outcome in death means that finding a way to prevent and treat it is urgent.

3
CAUSES OF ALZHEIMER'S DISEASE AND DEATH

Although scientists are still unsure what causes the brain to deteriorate in Alzheimer's disease, one of the longest-standing explanations of its mechanism focuses on the development of two injuries or lesions in the brain: plaques and tangles. In this chapter, I show how this mechanism of deterioration leads to the development of dementia, and later, how lithium can prevent and reverse this damage.

Plaques, Tangles, and Inflammation

Plaques form from deposits of small protein fragments called beta-amyloid peptides. Beta-amyloid, a byproduct of normal cellular activity, is usually cleared away by the cell's waste recycling processes. However, as we age, it can build up and form plaques. Clumps of these proteins block the spaces between neurons, or synapses. With the synapses barricaded, normal cell-to-cell signaling cannot occur, and communication stops. The physiological processes required for memory and learning halt, and symptoms develop. Moreover, the build-up of beta-amyloid peptides at cell junctions activates the immune system and triggers an inflammatory response. This further crowds the neurons and disrupts surrounding cells in other brain areas. Eventually, entire networks of neurons die and dissolve.[1]

While plaques form in the synapses between cells, other lesions, called neurofibrillary tangles, develop within the neurons themselves. These tangles result from a disruption in the production of a different type of protein called tau. Normally, tau protein filaments strengthen the small tubes that circulate nutrients and other essential supplies through the cell. When tau proteins function like they are supposed to, they act like the ties on railroad tracks—providing a structure that keeps trains running smoothly and the delivery of goods on schedule. In patients with Alzheimer's, however, tau proteins strands destabilize, becoming twisted, or "tangled." The tracks malfunction and eventually deteriorate. The system of transporting cell nutrients along the tracks is disrupted. Nutrients and other essential supplies can no longer move through the cells, which eventually die. Therefore, scientists think that the shrinkage of brain tissue in Alzheimer's disease results from three overlapping abnormal processes:

> Scientists think that the shrinkage of brain tissue in Alzheimer's disease results from 3 overlapping abnormal processes: beta-amyloid plaques, tau proteins and inflammation.

- Beta-amyloid plaques form between neurons, creating congestion and blocking communication.
- Tau proteins within nerve cells mutate and disrupt normal intracellular activity.
- Inflammatory cascades are triggered, further damaging and congesting surrounding tissues.

What Causes Plaques and Tangles?

In less than 5% of cases, Alzheimer's disease results from a specific genetic vulnerability that makes a person more likely to develop the disease. More often, plaques and tangles come from a complex combination of subtle genetic, lifestyle, and environmental factors that damage the brain over a lifetime. The brain can silently deteriorate over many years, even when memory and cognitive processes are still intact. This slow, cumulative development helps explain why most patients with Alzheimer's don't show signs or symptoms until after age 65.

Beta-amyloid plaques may be a relatively common malformation in the aging human brain, the iceberg below the surface. New research reveals that plaques may be present 30 to 40 years before symptoms of cognitive decline first appear.[2] Ten percent of 50-year-olds with intact mental skills have beta-amyloid deposits, according to one study.[1] The percentage of people whose brains have beta-amyloid deposits increases to 33% by age 80 and to 44% by age 90.[1]

> Most often, plaques and tangles come from a complex combination of subtle genetic, lifestyle, and environmental factors that damage the brain over a lifetime.

While it is common for people to develop some plaques and tangles as they age, people with Alzheimer's develop many more. As the disease progresses, the plaques and tangles form a predictable pattern, beginning in areas important in learning and memory and then spreading to other regions. Plaques generally precede tau tangles, and both are accompanied by inflammation in the brain and eventual neural loss.

Memory and cognitive ability depend on the clear and uninterrupted transmission of signals across one-hundred billion neurons. The plaques and tangles of Alzheimer's disease interfere with normal cell signal transmission and disrupt the activity of neurotransmitters, or chemical messengers. Scrambled chemistry produces flawed signaling, so the brain's messages—and with them, the ability to learn, remember, and communicate—are lost.

How Alzheimer's Leads to Death

Alzheimer's eventually causes death, but not directly. As neurons slowly di.e. your brain loses its functionality, which causes a cascading effect as it loses the ability to manage the intricate and complex bodily processes necessary to function first at a high level and then to function at all.

While the cause of death is Alzheimer's, the mechanism of death, or the actual organ damage or failure, is a different disease, or a complication of Alzheimer's. When basic motor functions such as swallowing and walking are disrupted, an Alzheimer's patient is at risk for secondary effects, including poor nutrition, dehydration, blood clots, falls, and infections. Such complications are called *intercurrent diseases* because they occur during the course of another disease.

> While the cause of patient death is Alzheimer's, the mechanism of death is usually a concurrent disease.

In people with advanced Alzheimer's, pneumonia is a leading cause of death, listed as the cause of death in as many as two-thirds of patients with dementia, according to the Alzheimer's Society. Lack of mobility diminishes the capacity of the lungs to expand and manage normal secretions properly, increasing susceptibility to pneumonia. The inability to swallow properly causes aspiration pneumonia, leading to damage or infection in the lungs that develops into pneumonia.

Other infections also frequently occur in people with advanced Alzheimer's, including urinary tract infections and serious skin infections, often due to ulcers or bed sores. Even when one infection is cured, it often comes back and eventually may not respond to antibiotic treatment.

Loss of interest in eating, difficulty swallowing, reduced capacity for self-feeding, and even the inability to express hunger or thirst to caregivers may lead Alzheimer's patients to not eat or drink enough for normal organ function. Dehydration and malnutrition can cause many serious and ultimately fatal problems, including inadequate heart function, reduced resistance to infection, bed sores, kidney failure, and coma.

> Older patients with Alzheimer's may have other life-threatening medical conditions that could be fatal even if they did not have Alzheimer's.

Older patients with Alzheimer's may have other life-threatening medical conditions, including chronic kidney disease, congestive heart failure, diabetes, coronary artery disease, stroke and cancer, that could be fatal even if they did not have Alzheimer's. Due to cognitive and behavioral changes, later-stage Alzheimer's patients are vulnerable to fatal accidents and injuries related to confusion and memory loss.

Summary

Many scientists believe that the brain atrophy observed in Alzheimer's disease results from three overlapping developments: beta-amyloid plaques, tau proteins, and inflammation. The damage develops slowly over time. These internal processes may begin decades before signs are visible.

Alzheimer's eventually causes death by intercurrent diseases, which intervene during the course of another disease. In people with advanced Alzheimer's, pneumonia is a leading cause of death. Other problems include urinary tract infections and serious skin infections. Dehydration and malnutrition can lead to inadequate heart function, reduced resistance to infection, bed sores, kidney failure, and coma.

Key Points

- Many experts believe that Alzheimer's is caused by clusters of beta-amyloid peptides that block the synapses and interfere with cell signaling. This occurs in combination with tangles in the neurons that disrupt transport of cell nutrients.
- Scientists now speculate that inflammation develops to clear the plaques and tangles and damages surrounding tissue.
- As the disease progresses, massive cell loss withers and shrinks the brain.
- While the cause of death is Alzheimer's, the mechanism of death— the actual damage or failure to the organs—is caused by a disease related to the Alzheimer's.

PART 2
THE SEARCH FOR RELIEF

4
DEAD-ENDS:
THE SEARCH FOR A DRUG CURE

This grim disease begs for a cure, yet finding effective treatment is tremendously complicated because scientists do not fully understand how it wields its damage. Most drugs focus on the familiar hypothesis that beta-amyloid plaques outside the cells and tau protein build-up inside the cells set up a cascade that ends in cell death. But medications to address the plaques and tangles directly have not been effective. Therefore, some scientists have suggested that beta-amyloid plaques may not be the primary cause of Alzheimer's but rather secondary effects. The failure of medications to affect beta-amyloid plaques has led researchers to pose other theories for the brain deterioration seen in Alzheimer's disease.

One proposed explanation is that the brains of people with Alzheimer's disease have low levels of acetylcholine, which is important for memory formation. Enzymes called cholinesterases break down acetylcholine. If their action is inhibited, more acetylcholine is presumably available for communication between brain cells. Based on this theory, some medicines marketed for Alzheimer's, including Aricept, manufactured by Pfizer, are cholinesterase inhibitors. They may help stabilize symptoms for a limited time but do not prevent disease

> One proposed explanation is that the brains of people with Alzheimer's disease have low levels of acetylcholine, which is important for memory formation.

progression. The three most commonly used cholinesterase inhibitors are donepezil (marketed as Aricept by Eisai), rivastigmine (Exelon, by Novartis Pharmaceuticals), and galantamine (Reminyl, by Janssen Pharmaceuticals). An earlier version, Tacrine (Cognex, by First Horizon Pharmaceutical), is no longer recommended due to its negative effects on the liver. In addition to not preventing disease progression, they can cause uncomfortable side effects such as dilation of the blood vessels; constriction of the pupils; increased secretion of sweat, saliva, and tears; slow heart rate; mucus secretion in the respiratory tract; and constriction of the airways.

Another theory attributes Alzheimer's to an aberration in the immune system that reacts with the beta-amyloid. Researchers at Northwestern University proposed that a smaller form of beta-amyloid, or oligomer, acts as a neurotoxin, adhering to cell receptors in the brain and jamming communication.[1] These oligomers may bind to a spot near a receptor in the hippocampus, called NMDA, which scientists believe helps establish new long-term memories. The NMDA receptor works like a tiny switch that permits ion signals to jump from cell to cell. The toxins attach to the receptor and keep the switch shut, disrupting cell-to-cell communication and, therefore, the creation of new memories. This communication is a key part of what neuroscientists call plasticity. So far, research based on this theory has produced no effective treatment.

> Another theory attributes Alzheimer's to an aberration in the immune system that reacts with the beta-amyloid.

A plethora of clinical trials have been launched in recent years, all with the goal of finding effective pharmacological interventions to stop or slow the progression of neurodegenerative disorders like Alzheimer's disease. However, from 2002 to 2012, fully 99.6% of drug

> What drugs are available may temporarily diminish Alzheimer's symptoms, none address the underlying mechanism of the disease.

studies aimed at preventing, curing, or mitigating Alzheimer's symptoms were either stopped or discontinued for lack of effectiveness.[2] Of 413 trials of proposed Alzheimer's drugs, only one drug made it to market.[2] Most of the tested drugs made patients sicker rather than better and came with disabling side effects. Patients and families in the midst of progressive dementia can find it difficult to decide if the risks are worth it, further adding to the confusion over the disease itself.

Despite years of clinical trials, currently, no medication is effective in preventing the progression of Alzheimer's disease. The available drugs, like Pfizer's Aricept and Namenda, a proprietary drug from Allergan, may temporarily improve symptoms but do not address the underlying disease mechanism. No new drugs have reached the market since 2001. This is certainly not because of lack of money or effort. Pharmaceutical companies are acutely aware that they would reap billions in profits if they could develop a drug that works, which is one reason these attempts have been consistent over the years. However, the history of clinical trials of Alzheimer's drugs is littered with failed attempts. In 2014, researchers found that, of 244 drugs studied for the treatment of Alzheimer's disease, only one was approved.[3] As a result, Alzheimer's drug candidates have one of the highest failure rates of any disease, at 99.6%—compared with 81% for cancer.[3] Recently, Merck discontinued its Phase III trial of verubecestat, which had appeared to have potential earlier in the clinical trial process.[4] The 1,958 patients who had taken the study drug eventually had no better cognitive outcomes than the study subjects on placebo. For ethical reasons, Merck terminated the trial.

The pharmaceutical industry remains highly committed to developing expensive, patentable drugs for dementia and Alzheimer's disease. The prospect of enormous profit continues to drive this experimentation. The ability of companies to advertise Alzheimer's disease medications directly to families rather than to physicians and healthcare professionals only adds to the public confusion about efficacy and the risk of widespread use of ineffective treatments.

Earlier Intervention

However, recently, the race to find a cure has shifted. Recent studies suggest that research to find a drug to reverse Alzheimer's has focused on an intervention point too late in the disease course. Many researchers have now shifted efforts away from treating late-stage Alzheimer's disease, when, to date, deterioration of the brain has been shown to be irreversible. Instead, they have recognized the need to aim for an earlier intervention point. New evidence that plaques begin to build up in the brain years before signs and symptoms of cognitive decline appear suggests that expending all research resources on treatment of a longstanding illness makes little sense. By the time a diagnosis of Alzheimer's is confirmed with current screening techniques, the internal damage is substantial and mostly beyond the reach of pharmaceuticals.

In a 2012 paper, "Why have we failed to cure Alzheimer's Disease?", Korczyn wrote:

> Attempts to find cures for Alzheimer's disease have. . . failed so far, in spite of enormous investments, intellectual and financial. We therefore have to reconsider the problem from new angles. Alzheimer's is regarded as a disease because of its clinical manifestations and underlying pathology. However, this combination does not define a disease but rather a syndrome. . . It is probable that senile dementia is the result of a combination of several processes, working differently in each person. Thus, a concerted action to fight the dementia epidemic must be made by aggressive action against its risk factors, and this battle must begin in midlife, not in old age.[5]

This revelation has been extremely important not just in my own clinical practice but in the greater understanding of where the puzzle piece of dementia prevention fits. For now, it's important to recognize that risk factors themselves are being identified, allowing room for preventive intervention. After so many failed pharmaceutical attempts to stop the degenerative process of late-stage Alzheimer's disease, considerable attention is now focused on an earlier window of time as a target. Researchers and clinicians have recognized the need to find a therapy to strengthen and protect the brain from damage and prevent the formation of plaques and tangles before they impair memory and behavior.

> After so many failed pharmaceutical attempts to stop the degenerative process of late-stage Alzheimer's disease, considerable attention is now focused on an earlier window of time as a target.

The optimal solution would be safe, affordable, and effective and would have both neuroprotective and neurogenerative abilities.

Biotechnical companies have raised billions of dollars in attempts to find a preventive neuroprotective treatment. Most of their efforts have been futile. With so many individuals and families suffering, both the stakes and the investments are high. Yet while precious dollars from governments, charity organizations, and generous donors are gambled away on these trials, scientific literature has already clearly identified a preventive strategy that works. The only problem is that it isn't patentable and therefore isn't profitable. The financial incentive to establish and conduct scientific trials is minimal, yet the potential for relief from the scourge of the twenty-first century is immeasurable. As you will learn in the next chapter, this strategy was discovered by accident.

Summary

The failure of all medications for Alzheimer's disease to date stems from scientists' inability to fully understand the mechanisms of the disease. Medications to directly affect plaques and tangles have not been effective, which has led researchers to propose other mechanisms for Alzheimer's.

Hundreds of drug trials have been launched in the past 30 years to find effective treatments. As pharmaceutical investigators have abandoned contenders that seemed promising but proved ineffective, some scientists have shifted their focus from trying to treat late-stage Alzheimer's to targeting an earlier intervention point. It appears that by the time the diagnosis of Alzheimer's disease is confirmed, internal damage is severe and probably irreversible.

Key Points

- Failure of drugs to directly eradicate plaques and tangles has led to alternative hypotheses of the disease mechanisms behind Alzheimer's disease.
- One proposed explanation for Alzheimer's disease is low levels of acetylcholine, which is essential for memory. Cholinesterases are enzymes that break down acetylcholine. Drugs like Pfizer's Aricept inhibit cholinesterase but do not prevent Alzheimer's progression.
- Pharmaceutical trials for Alzheimer's drugs have all failed to identify an effective drug.
- Recent research tends to target an earlier intervention point and multiple pathways that may contribute to the disease process.

5
AN ACCIDENTAL DISCOVERY: LITHIUM

Now we must turn from the debacle of dead-end pharmaceutical trials to research into the benefits of a simple element for treating another problem. For many years, scientists have known that the simple mineral lithium keeps neurons healthy. It has long been the first-line treatment for bipolar disorder and one of the best augmentive treatments for depression. I have been treating psychiatric patients with therapeutic doses of lithium for more than three decades.

In fact, the benefits of lithium for treating bipolar disorder have been known since 1952, when Erik Stromgren, head of the Aarhus University Psychiatric Clinic in Risskov, Denmark, encouraged staff psychiatrist Mogens Schou to design and conduct what turned out to be one of the first randomized controlled trials in the history of medicine.[1] The trial compared lithium with a placebo in treating patients

> When a trial concluded that lithium was effective as an alternative to electroconvulsive therapy, some medical professionals began to regard this mineral as nothing short of a miracle.

with manic depression, or bipolar disorder. When the trial concluded that lithium was effective as an alternative to electroconvulsive therapy, some medical professionals began to regard this mineral as nothing short of a miracle.

In the United States, rigorous studies of lithium during the 1960s concluded that it was effective in treating both the manic and depressive phases of bipolar disorder. Over the next several decades, hundreds of studies confirmed that lithium improved symptoms of various mental conditions, including depression, that had been difficult to treat. Every so often, a pharmaceutical company's proprietary drug intended for bipolar disorder was introduced to the market with a lavish launch, and lithium's bright light briefly dimmed. Eventually, though, lithium retained its steadfast superiority over other medications, and it became the gold standard for treating bipolar disorder.

In October 2000, a research team at Wayne State University School of Medicine made an accidental discovery while studying lithium's mechanism of action in bipolar disorder.[2] They found that, in addition to stabilizing mood, this remarkable mineral protects brain cells from premature death. They reported that lithium might even cause brain cells to regenerate after loss from disease.

The researchers posited that lithium works by increasing a good protein in the brain while decreasing a bad one.[2] It increases concentrations of a gene that protects brain cells from ionizing radiation while decreasing levels of a protein that spurs the production of neurofibrillary tangles. The scientists were surprised when they examined the magnetic resonance imaging (MRI) scans of the brains of study subjects treated with lithium because they found something they had not been looking for: the gray matter in the brains of bipolar patients on lithium had actually increased.[3] These scans revealed clear evidence that contradicted accepted wisdom that the phenomenon of nerve cell creation, or neurogenesis, occurs exclusively in the early stages of life. Scientists had long thought the adult brain could only lose cells, not gain them. But here were clear images that constituted undeniable evidence: adult brains were regenerating cells.

> Scientists had long thought the adult brain could only lose cells, not gain them. But here were clear images that constituted undeniable evidence: adult brains were regenerating cells.

Turning their attention from bipolar disorder, the researchers conducted an in vitro study to test lithium's influence on brain cell survival. They incubated human brain cells in a lithium solution and exposed them to two different toxins.[3] The cells that had been treated with lithium had an astonishing 220% higher survival rate than cells in the control group, which had not been treated with lithium. The Wayne State team reasoned that because Alzheimer's disease results from cell death, lithium's potential in preventing Alzheimer's would be a fruitful area for research.[3]

Although studies demonstrating the neuroprotective potential of lithium have appeared in the scientific literature for decades, this was the first time lithium's potential was explicitly linked to the prevention of cognitive decline.

> Long considered a gold standard for the treatment of bipolar disorder, lithium is lately attracting attention for its remarkable neuroprotective properties.

Subsequent studies support the Wayne State researchers' findings. Large research trials of lithium's effects have shown that patients treated with lithium for bipolar disorder have a lower incidence of Alzheimer's disease than the general population. In a study of 6,900 older adults with bipolar disorder, prescribed lithium appeared to decrease dementia risk by 23%.[4]

Attempting to better understand this link, a group of researchers compared the rates of Alzheimer's disease in 66 elderly bipolar patients on long-term lithium therapy with 48 similar patients not taking lithium. The differences were impressive: in patients receiving continuous lithium, the prevalence of Alzheimer's was 5%, compared with 33% in the control group.[5] Two studies in Denmark confirmed this phenomenon using different study designs but yielding strikingly similar results.[6] In this series, investigators surveyed the records of more than 21,000 patients who had received lithium treatment. They found that lithium was associated with decreased rates of both dementia in general and Alzheimer's disease in particular.[6]

Individual studies of lithium treatment for bipolar patients have identified specific cognitive benefits of the treatment. Those treated with lithium demonstrate better visual memory than counterparts not taking lithium.[7]

Lithium may be most effective in prevention and treatment of early Alzheimer's disease when used at microdose or supplemental levels, similar to those found naturally in water and foods. In a study published in *Alzheimer's Research*, a tiny dose of 0.3 mg lithium was administered once daily to Alzheimer's patients for 15 months.[8] They had stable results on cognitive performance tests throughout the study, while the results of cognitive tests in the control group demonstrated progressive decline. In addition, three months into the study, the seemingly impossible occurred: the patients with Alzheimer's got better.[8] Those treated with lithium scored higher on standardized assessments of cognitive function than they had scored before the study began.

> Lithium may be most effective in preventing and treating early Alzheimer's disease when used at micro-dose or supplemental levels.

These positive research results of low-dose lithium effectiveness followed four large studies of the effects of lithium in tap water, conducted in the United States, Denmark, and Japan. Each study confirmed an association between lithium at trace doses in drinking water and low levels of Alzheimer's disease and dementia. A large study conducted in 2017 in Denmark matched the cases of 73,731 patients with dementia and 733,653 controls according to the presence or absence of lithium in their local water supply.[9] Those whose water contained lithium had lower rates of dementia than controls. A 2018 article in the *Journal of Alzheimer's Disease* concluded that lithium in drinking water is linked to longer life in patients with Alzheimer's.[10]

> The positive effects that lithium caused were not found in studies assessing the benefits of anticonvulsants, antidepressants, or antipsychotic drugs.

After completing a meta-analysis of many studies exploring a link between lithium and Alzheimer's treatment, Matsanaga found that across the studies, lithium improved cognitive performance in patients with mild cognitive impairment and Alzheimer's disease.[11] In general, improvement in patients' cognitive function was inversely related to the severity of dementia symptoms. The positive effects of lithium were not found in studies assessing the benefits of anticonvulsants, antidepressants, or antipsychotic drugs.[11]

To date, then, a drug used in higher doses to treat patients with bipolar disorder has turned out to slow and even reverse the devastating effects of Alzheimer's. The researchers at Wayne State, who were trying to understand lithium's mechanism of action against bipolar disease, happened to see unexpected results. Then they had the foresight to realize their discovery would lead to a promising new line of inquiry.

Summary

Lithium's neuroprotective capacity has been known to scientists for many years. Used since the 1950s for treating bipolar disorder, it is now the gold standard treatment for this mood disorder. In 2000, researchers made an accidental, fortuitous discovery. They realized that lithium, in addition to stabilizing mood, protects brain cells from premature death. Subsequently, MRI studies revealed that lithium can increase gray matter in the brain. Because dementia results from brain cell death, the researchers hypothesized that lithium could be useful in treating Alzheimer's disease.

The researchers observed that the dementia rate was lower in bipolar patients treated with lithium than in the general population. In patients without bipolar disorder, microdose lithium improved the cognitive function of Alzheimer's patients. Studies also showed that rates of Alzheimer's disease are lower in regions where lithium is added to drinking water.

Key Points

- Lithium has been used successfully to treat bipolar disease since the 1950s.
- Although many medications for bipolar disorder have been launched since that time, lithium remains the gold standard treatment.

- Researchers at Wayne State University discovered in 2000 that lithium protects against cell death and even leads to regeneration of gray matter.
- Lithium protects against Alzheimer's disease at microdose levels.
- Large analyses in Texas, Denmark, and Japan show that the Alzheimer's rate in areas that have drinking water treated with lithium is lower than in untreated areas.

PART 3
LITHIUM AND
ALZHEIMER'S DISEASE

6
MINERALS AND TOXICITY: LITHIUM IN CONTEXT

In order to understand how low-dose lithium fits into the bigger picture of integrative psychiatry, it's important to have some context on nutritional interventions in general. To sustain life, your body must have a wide variety of nutrients, many of which include trace amounts of many common minerals such as calcium and magnesium. They are essential for human livelihood, maintaining homeostasis, and basic physiological processes. However, all of these vital nutrients also have toxic levels—when too much is ingested, they become dangerous. As Swiss alchemist and physician Paracelsus (1493–1541) said almost five-hundred years ago, "All substances are poisons; there is none that is not a poison. The right dose differentiates a poison from a remedy."

The truth is that hundreds of substances are not only beneficial but necessary at low doses but toxic at high doses. All chemicals, from whatever source, natural or manufactured, are potentially toxic at some dose. This fundamental concept underlies toxicology and is critical to the assessment of risk from chemicals and their safe use. The concept is the dose-response relationship—the amount of the substance that causes

> Only a skewed understanding of the dose-response relationship would lead someone to forgo the benefits of low-dose lithium because it is toxic in high doses.

it to be toxic—not the substance itself. The degree to which a substance is toxic is related to the dose-time relationship, exposure route, gender, weight, condition, age, and the ability of a substance to be absorbed, distributed, metabolized, and finally excreted from the body. For example, faster absorption and/or slower excretion may suggest greater toxicity. This relationship depends on the properties of the substance itself and the characteristics of the person ingesting it.

Here are some minerals that in small amounts are necessary to life but that are toxic when too much is ingested. Scientists generally classify them into two groups: the seven macro minerals and the many minerals you need in trace amounts.

Seven Macro Minerals

Calcium is required to build and maintain strong bones. It is also needed by the heart, muscles, and nerves. Along with vitamin D, it may protect against cancer, diabetes, and high blood pressure. Calcium deficiency increases the risk of osteoporosis, osteopenia, and hypocalcemia. But in large amounts, calcium is bad for you. Overdoses can lead to stomachache, constipation or diarrhea, headache, nausea, and vomiting. High levels of calcium in the body, called hypercalcemia, can lead to anorexia and to severe cardiac problems.

Chlorine is essential for all life species. Located in all body fluids, it transmits nerve impulses, maintains a balance between acids and bases, and regulates fluid in and out of cells. It is also a key element in metabolism. Ingesting too much chlorine, however, can cause severe symptoms. It can irritate the gastrointestinal tract and even lead to respiratory distress, convulsions and, rarely, death.

Magnesium is critical to nerve transmission, muscle contraction, blood coagulation, energy production, nutrient metabolism, and bone and cell formation. It activates more than three-hundred enzyme reactions in the body, which translate to thousands of biochemical reactions throughout the day. Too much magnesium, typically consumed through laxatives and antacids providing more than 5,000 mg/day, can cause weakness, confusion, decreased breathing rate, and dizziness. In very high doses, magnesium can lead to cardiac arrest.

Phosphorus is a mineral required for strong bones and teeth. It also helps store and use energy and support growth. Too much phosphorus causes joint and muscle pain and gastrointestinal distress.

Potassium is an essential mineral that supports cardiac and tissue health and gastrointestinal function. It helps decrease risk of stroke, cardiovascular disease, osteoporosis, kidney stones, and high blood pressure. But abnormally high levels of potassium incite muscular weakness, temporary paralysis, and cardiac arrhythmia.

Sodium is an essential mineral that sends nerve impulses throughout our bodies and regulates fluid balance. Too little sodium can lead to mental changes, seizures, and even coma and death. However, too much sodium is also harmful, causing water retention, which can lead to high blood pressure. This in turn places greater strain on the heart, arteries, kidneys, and brain.

Sulfur, the third most abundant mineral in the body, is essential for amino acids that create protein for cells, tissues, hormones, enzymes, and antibodies. A deficiency of sulfur can cause or exacerbate conditions such as arthritis, chronic fatigue, depression, heart disease, memory loss, and slow wound healing. Too much sulfur can irritate the gastrointestinal system, respiratory system, and the skin and eyes.

Trace Minerals

In addition to these seven macro minerals, the body needs many trace minerals, including iron, selenium, chromium, cobalt, copper, fluorine, iodine, molybdenum, and zinc. Similar to the seven macro minerals, all of them are necessary for life and are toxic when ingested in excessive amounts. In this context, you can see that only a skewed understanding of the dose-response relationship would lead someone to forgo the benefits of low-dose lithium because it is toxic in high doses.

Lithium has undergone a shifting and dramatic history in medicine, sometimes celebrated as a panacea, sometimes reviled as toxic, sometimes totally forgotten before reappearing in scientific experiments in another country in another context. Still, after the intervening centuries and billion-dollar pharmaceutical efforts, no drug has superseded lithium for preventing cognitive decline and degeneration of Alzheimer's disease. Currently, the most promising intervention to protect against brain atrophy is psychiatry's oldest medication, which is simply a mineral essential for brain health.

> Still, after the intervening centuries and billion-dollar pharmaceutical efforts, no drug has superseded lithium for preventing the degeneration of Alzheimer's disease.

Summary

All substances are toxic at certain doses, including the minerals and nutrients that sustain life and maintain homeostasis. The dose-response relationship—the amount of a substance that causes it to be toxic—is determined by the method of exposure; the individual's weight, condition, and age; and the ability of a substance to be absorbed, distributed, metabolized, and finally excreted from the body. Substances like calcium, magnesium, and lithium can be therapeutic at low doses and toxic at high ones.

Key Points

- To understand low-dose lithium and toxicity, we must contextualize mineral toxicity as a whole.
- Minerals like calcium and magnesium are vital for human life but toxic at high levels.
- A misunderstanding may cause some to forgo the benefits of low-dose lithium because it is toxic in high doses.

7
THE HISTORY OF LITHIUM IN MEDICINE

Medical use of lithium was first publicized by London doctor Alfred Baring Garrod in treating patients with gout, a form of arthritis characterized by inflammation and hardened deposits that cause pain in the joints. Garrod publicized the lithium treatment of gout—including "brain gout"— through his 1859 work, *The Nature and Treatment of Gout and Rheumatic Gout*. The Sears, Roebuck & Company Catalogue of 1908 advertised Schieffelin's Effervescent Lithia Tablets for a variety of afflictions. By 1907, The *Merck Index* listed 43 different medicinal preparations containing lithium. Excitement about these products reflected the predominant view that uric acid causes a plethora of diseases and negative outcomes, including headache, epilepsy, depression, melancholia, suicide, high blood pressure, angina, asthma, Raynaud's disease, gout, and rheumatism. As the popularity of the uric acid explanation for disease declined, interest in lithium products waned.[1]

Psychiatric applications of lithium began in 1870, when Philadelphia neurologist Silas Weir Mitchell recommended lithium bromide as an anticonvulsant and hypnotic and later for "general nervousness."[2] The next year, William Hammond, professor of diseases of the mind and nervous system at Bellevue Hospital Medical College in New York, became the first physician to prescribe lithium for mania.

Lithium was first seriously used to treat mood disorders in Denmark. Two psychiatrist brothers, Fredrik and Carl Lange, reported in the first Danish textbook of clinical psychiatry that they had successfully used lithium in patients with depression.[3] After the brothers' death, however, the potential of lithium in treating mood disorders was forgotten. The twentieth century revival of lithium as a psychiatric remedy began in 1949 with John Cade, who designed a well-structured research study that concluded that lithium helped patients with bipolar disorder, even those who had been ill for years and had been unsuccessfully treated with other medications.[4] Cade knew of Alfred Garrod's success in using lithium a century before for gout. He hypothesized that a condition involving uric acid might underlie the behavior of his manic patients; he speculated that they had a metabolic disorder, indicated by excessive urea in their urine.

Cade tested his theory by injecting uric acid into guinea pigs. To make an injectable solution, he used lithium urate for the simple reason that it was highly soluble. To Cade's surprise, the treatment produced a calming effect instead of increased excitation. Through a series of very careful experiments on both guinea pigs and human subjects, he proved that lithium had a pronounced calming effect on mania. Cade began treating patients with lithium citrate and lithium carbonate. Some responded remarkably well, becoming essentially normal and capable of leaving the hospital after years of illness. Cade presented his research results in a rational tone rather than rhapsodizing about the virtues of a particular treatment. Because of his well-designed studies and their dramatic results, some historians of medicine believe that John Cade ushered in the field of psychopharmacology.

The timing of Cade's treatment success was unfortunate, however. The very same year, 1949, adverse reaction reports surfaced in the media about patients taking lithium in a different form for a completely different purpose. As physicians began to encourage their heart patients to avoid sodium chloride, lithium chloride was marketed as an alternative. Some patients developed lithium poisoning after consuming large amounts of lithium chloride. Several

> Careless inattention to regulating dosages of lithium has led the medical establishment to become skeptical of lithium, a reluctance that continues to this day.

deaths were reported, leading the U.S. Food and Drug Administration (FDA) to ban lithium salt substitutes. "Stop using this dangerous poison at once!" exhorted the FDA. Unsurprisingly, lithium fell out of favor with the medical community.[1] This careless inattention to regulating lithium doses led the medical establishment to become skeptical about the use of lithium, a reluctance that continues to this day.

Despite the lithium chloride debacle, Cade's study prompted a few isolated studies of lithium in Australia and France. The next breakthrough happened again in Denmark. Psychiatrist Mogens Schou tried an entirely new research design: a randomized controlled trial.[5] This experiment would study the effectiveness of lithium for treating bipolar disorder by randomly assigning patients—literally by tossing a coin—to receive either lithium or placebo. Schou's experiment revealed that 70% of patients responded to lithium.[5] Schou introduced the term "mood normalizer" to convey lithium's ability to stabilize abnormal mood swings while not affecting normal emotions in the ways that amphetamines and barbiturates do. Charting the natural history of bipolar disorder, with its predictable recurrences and progressive character, he demonstrated lithium's beneficial effects not only as a maintenance drug but also as a preventive medication.[2]

The United States was slow to embrace and fund the study of lithium. But gradually, a "lithium underground" formed of physicians prescribing lithium in the absence of official FDA approval. Finally, in 1970, the United States was the fiftieth country to approve lithium for treatment of acute mania. Later, it was also approved to prevent recurrent mania.

> The United States was slow to embrace and fund the study of lithium. But gradually, a "lithium underground" formed of physicians prescribing lithium in the absence of official FDA approval.

There followed an upsurge in prescriptions for lithium to treat patients for acute mania and prevent relapse of both manic and depressive cycles in bipolar disorder. Lithium was established as the gold standard treatment for bipolar disorder. When newer, more expensive medications were launched with extravagant advertising, lithium temporarily lost its place as the first-line treatment for bipolar disorder. An undercurrent of skepticism remained, mostly because lithium in high doses had proved toxic.

Summary

Lithium was first used medically to treat gout. Later, John Cade popularized the use of lithium citrate and lithium carbonate for mood disorders with his study that concluded that these forms of lithium helped patients with bipolar disorder. Some consider his work the birth of psychopharmacology.

Due to public distrust of other forms of lithium, which in high doses lead to lithium poisoning, lithium fell out of favor with the medical community. However, research continued internationally. Research in Australia, Denmark, and France led to further acceptance of lithium as an effective treatment for mood disorders, including bipolar, though the United States was slow to catch on again. Finally, in 1970, the United States was the fiftieth country to approve lithium for the treatment of acute mania.

Key Points

- Though it showed promise early on, lithium research and treatment was stalled after widespread distrust in the medical community of all forms of lithium.
- Inattention to the variance in form and dosage led to a lack of interest.
- It has been scientifically demonstrated in several countries that low-dose lithium can be therapeutic in Alzheimer's disease.
- Research continued abroad, and slowly the United States began to accept and understand the use of lithium for mood disorders, and now, for an abundance of health benefits.

8
THE CINDERELLA DRUG:
WHY WE'RE SLOW TO RECOGNIZE
LITHIUM'S VALUE

Cornell psychiatrist Anna Fels calls lithium a "Cinderella drug" because, despite its clearly demonstrated value, it is neglected and ignored.[1] Though early promise turned to doubt and skepticism, a slow movement has emerged towards embracing lithium once again. Lithium is safe and inexpensive, has shown years of promise through clinical trials and research, and seems to answer many questions about how to prevent dementia and keep our brains healthy. So why is it not used more widely? I think there are several reasons.

No Financial Incentive

The most obvious is that lithium is simple and inexpensive. Although the potential for relief from brain deterioration is enormous, there is little financial incentive for research on lithium. Companies are not interested in developing a new pitch for an old drug. Instead, they fund research studies to test drugs that will generate profit. The sophisticated, glossy advertisements

> Some scientists call lithium a "Cinderella drug" because, despite its clearly demonstrated value, it is widely neglected and ignored.

that come across a doctor's desk or on TV commercials trumpet drugs that will enrich the pharmaceutical company. These companies have nothing to gain by researching or marketing an inexpensive element that is available everywhere and is not patentable. Lithium lacks the excitement of novelty and the fanfare of an extravagant launch.

Stigma of Association with Mental Illness

Perhaps another reason that physicians are slow to consider lithium for their patients with cognitive decline is the stigma sometimes associated with the drug. Physicians may hesitate to prescribe lithium based on its connection with bipolar disorder and the stigma of mental health treatment. Lithium may also be slow to catch on because of its reputation as the cause of serious side effects in earlier decades. For lithium doses generally prescribed today, this blame is misplaced and the reputation undeserved.

> Perhaps another reason that physicians are slow to consider lithium for their patients with cognitive decline is the stigma sometimes associated with the drug.

The perception that lithium is a dangerous drug may also be a residual effect based on some patients' experiences from the 1960s to the 1980s. During this period, physicians sometimes prescribed high doses of lithium that eventually led to serious side effects, including kidney problems and even kidney failure. Today's recommended dosages are much lower to prevent patients from developing side effects. The reputation of lithium as a dangerous drug may linger even though it is no longer accurate. The safety of lithium is particularly striking when it is used for Alzheimer's disease, as microdoses of the mineral appear to be most helpful for slowing cognitive decline.

The Tomato Effect

A phenomenon called the "tomato effect" may also help explain why the medical community is slow to recognize the clear benefits of a therapy like lithium that has been around for a long time. The tomato effect was identified by Drs. James and Jean Goodwin in 1984 in the *Journal of the American Medical Association*.[2] They wrote, "The tomato effect in medicine occurs when an efficacious treatment for a certain disease is ignored or rejected because it does not 'make sense' in light of accepted theories of disease mechanism and drug action."

The rejection of a potentially useful treatment because "everyone knows it won't work" is named for Americans' stubborn belief—from the sixteenth to the nineteenth centuries—that tomatoes were poisonous. Although tomatoes were first eaten in the Americas, they were viewed as inedible decorative plants in the 1600s and 1700s. They were believed to be poisonous because they belong to the nightshade family of plants, of which belladonna and mandrake are indeed toxic. But Americans also knew that Europeans were serving and eating tomatoes at the dinner table.

The fate of the tomato in the United States changed in 1820, when a man named Robert Johnson of Salem, NJ, consumed a basketful of tomatoes in public to prove they were safe to eat. When he neither dropped dead nor suffered any apparent ill effects, the witnesses to his experiment slowly began to open their minds. By the end of the decade, American gardeners in the Northeast were growing tomatoes for food.

Understanding this human tendency to reject a treatment outside of one's usual frame of reference—even

> Understanding this human tendency to reject a treatment outside of one's usual frame of reference—even in the face of contradictory evidence—helps explain how slow many researchers have been to pay attention to the amazing potential of lithium.

in the face of contradictory evidence—helps explain how slow many researchers have been to pay attention to the amazing potential of lithium.

Disappointing Results of Early Research Trials

Finally, lithium may be slow to gain favor because the first clinical trials designed to test the mineral with dementia patients yielded disappointing results. Researchers first attempted to fit lithium into the same framework used by drug companies: testing patients who already had fully developed Alzheimer's disease. At this point, damage to the brain was too great to reverse.

> Lithium may be slow to gain favor because the first clinical trials designed to test the mineral with dementia patients yielded disappointing results.

Several studies concluded that lithium was not effective against late-stage Alzheimer's disease. One small, open-label study looked at low-dose lithium use in 22 Alzheimer's patients over one year.[3] These patients had advanced cognitive decline secondary to Alzheimer's disease. While researchers concluded that lithium was safe in this population, no cognitive benefits were observed in the patients. It is now clear that the intervention was too late to make a difference in the advanced stages of illness, when plaques and neurofibrillary tangles are already embedded in the neuronal architecture.

Another study yielded disappointing results for a different reason. This multicenter study explored the use of lithium sulfate in participants with mild Alzheimer's over a 10-week period.[4] No significant effects of lithium treatment on cognitive performance or related biomarkers were observed. The major problem with this trial, however, was its length. It takes months, not weeks, to see substantial cognitive shifts in patients who have developed a disease over a span of 40 years.

Forlenza and colleagues attempted to correct for these initial design flaws. Focusing on prevention rather than treatment of already developed Alzheimer's disease, they designed a study to assess whether long-term lithium treatment could prevent Alzheimer's in high-risk individuals.[5] Forty-five participants with mild cognitive impairment, a precursor to Alzheimer's, were randomly assigned to receive lithium or a placebo. Over the 12-month trial, lithium dosages were kept at subtherapeutic levels (150 to 600 mg daily) to minimize potential side effects.

This time, results were promising. Fewer destructive tau proteins were present in the brains of lithium-treated patients after the study. In the placebo group, on the other hand, tau levels had increased steadily.[5] Moreover, the lithium group showed improved performance on multiple cognitive scales. The patients tolerated the lithium well, as there were few reported side effects, and patients' adherence to treatment was impressive (91%). Researchers concluded from the study that lithium helps prevent dementia and Alzheimer's disease when initiated early in the disease progression.

We now know that the dangerous plaques and tangles that debilitate the Alzheimer's brain start as many as 40 years before signs and symptoms appear. Ten percent of healthy 50 year olds already have amyloid deposits in their brain tissues. For

> "If lithium prevents dementia, then we may have overlooked a very simple means of preventing a major public health problem."
> ~Dr. Nassir Ghaemi

optimal effectiveness, steps to protect the brain must be taken at a much younger age than previously thought. When started early, low-dose lithium may be the key intervention to prevent cognitive decline. By shifting the target point from late treatment to prevention, these interventions highlight the exciting potential of lithium for not only stopping ongoing deterioration in dementia but even for encouraging cognitive repair early in treatment.

Dr. Nassir Ghaemi, professor of psychiatry at Tufts University Medical School, concluded, "Lithium is, by far, the most proven drug to keep neurons alive, in animals and in humans, consistently and with many replicated studies. If lithium prevents dementia, then we may have overlooked a very simple means of preventing a major public health problem."[1]

> But now it is time for the medical community to inform Alzheimer's sufferers and their families—as well as patients who wish to avoid future brain cell deterioration—that a critical nutritional intervention is already available.

Many factors may combine to explain why lithium has been overlooked. But now it is time for the medical community to inform Alzheimer's sufferers and their families—as well as patients who wish to avoid future brain cell deterioration—that a critical nutritional intervention is already available. It is not a costly new drug but an ordinary, naturally occurring mineral in water, rocks, and soil since ancient times.

Summary

Several reasons help explain why the medical and scientific communities have been slow to recognize the value of lithium. Because lithium is a mineral that occurs in nature, there is no financial incentive to support research trials and no expectation of profit from manufacture. Moreover, because of lithium's association with treatment of bipolar disease, the stigma of mental illness may prevent some physicians from recommending lithium and some individuals from taking it. The human tendency to reject a treatment outside the usual frame of reference is another possible reason lithium is underused. Finally, the results of early clinical trials of lithium for Alzheimer's disease were disappointing. Since that time, researchers have learned that lithium confers its benefits when administered early in the disease process.

Key Points

- Drug companies have nothing to gain by researching or marketing lithium.
- Lithium's association with treatment of mood disorders may deter both physicians and patients with cognitive decline from using it.
- Recent studies have shown that lithium can reduce plaques and tangles in the brain and foster improved cognitive performance in patients with mild cognitive impairment or early Alzheimer's disease.

9
HOW LITHIUM PROTECTS
AGAINST ALZHEIMER'S

Since the discovery that lithium can protect brain cells from deterioration and even spur cell regeneration, we know more about how lithium works in Alzheimer's disease.

The blossoming of the nervous system from a simple cell to the sophisticated biochemical framework that houses our thoughts, emotions, and drive for survival is a miracle of human life. We used to believe that nerve cell creation, or neurogenesis, occurred only in early life. The brain grows four times its size during the preschool period, reaching about 90% of adult size by age six. After that, we thought, brain cell growth lessens.

Studies using MRI techniques gave us the first hard evidence that lithium promotes cell growth. Researchers studied the brain volume of 12 bipolar patients taking lithium to regulate mood.[1] They were shocked by what they found: patients taking lithium had significantly more total gray matter than bipolar patients not taking lithium. Another study focused on lithium's effects on the hippocampus, an area of the brain involved in emotion and memory.[2] Results were similar: the hippocampus was 14% larger in lithium-treated patients than in those not taking lithium. At least three other studies have had these same results.[3]

> The researchers were shocked: patients taking lithium had significantly more total gray matter than bipolar patients not taking lithium.

This new awareness has dizzying implications for our understanding of neurodegenerative diseases. Scientists used to think that the brain and nervous system had only a certain number of cells, and any damage to them was permanent, devastating, and irreversible. This image of the brain as fixed and stagnant meant that anyone with a neurological illness had a grim prognosis. This idea also led to a dismal outlook on aging, as brain cells undergo wear and tear over time.

> The scientifically established fact that lithium fosters neuroprotection and neurogenesis has exciting implications for the aging brain: brain shrinkage and brain cell loss can be reversed.

We thought that brains shrunk and cells died because they were the unavoidable results of aging, like gray hair and wrinkles. These recent studies, however, have shown us we were wrong. Although most neurons appear before birth, neurons and their connections can grow over a lifetime, depending on the availability of nutritional building blocks like amino acids, fatty acids, essential vitamins —and minerals like lithium.

Lithium Enhances Cell Growth and Neuroprotection

Lithium helps cells grow in specific ways. Neurotrophic factors are proteins that regulate the growth and survival of neurons. Lithium stimulates the circulation of several key neurotrophic factors.[4-6] One neurotropic factor helps nervous system cells grow, mature, and maintain. It is found mostly in the synapses, or spaces between neurons, where it promotes cell-to-cell communication and signaling. Nerve cell synapses can strengthen and weaken over time in response to experiences, a process called synaptic plasticity. Lithium also regulates synaptic plasticity, an important biochemical underpinning of learning and memory.

Lithium Increases Nerve Cell Function

Lithium increases concentrations of a key chemical called N-acetyl-aspartate (NAA) in the brain. It is considered a marker of neuronal wellness, with high levels showing increased brain cell function and viability.[7] At least 20 studies have explored how NAA works in brain disease, concluding that higher NAA levels predict better long-term brain function.[8,9]

> At the cellular level, lithium exerts powerful influences on neuroprotection and brain health, thus protecting against changes associated with Alzheimer's disease through a variety of pathways.

Several studies have shown that lithium safely and effectively raises NAA levels in people of all ages. One study evaluated lithium treatment and NAA levels in older adults. Although the study sample was small, researchers found promising evidence that lithium promoted healthy brain tissue development in older people.[9]

Lithium Regulates Key Enzymes

Lithium regulates the enzyme glycogen-synthase kinase-3 (GSK3). This unique enzyme acts on more than 40 different proteins in the body. In the nervous system, GSK3 helps neurons grow and develop by activating proteins in the cells, driving memory formation. It helps signal when excess or old neurons should die. Ordinarily, this is a healthy process because the brain needs to rid itself of waste. On the other hand, in many brain diseases, the process is too much, too quickly.[10,11]

Tight regulation of GSK3 ensures that healthy signaling pathways are maintained in mature brain tissue. Overactivity of GSK3 in the brain areas that control memory and behavior leads to production of proteins such as beta-amyloid and tau proteins at too rapid a rate. They build up, creating plaques and tangles.

Researchers are searching for ways to inhibit GSK3. Fortunately, lithium is a well-established GSK3 inhibitor. By dimming GSK3 activity, lithium slows the production of beta-amyloid and tau proteins and prevents related damage.[11-13] In a 2016 study, fruit flies treated with low-dose lithium to target GSK3 lived longer, independent of other factors like genetic background and sex. The researchers said that lithium can lengthen life and shorten physical and mental decline the end of life. The researchers' next step is to target GSK3 in more complex animals, with the goal of human testing.[14]

Lithium Removes Plaques and Tangles from Cells

In addition to slowing beta-amyloid and tau protein production, lithium promotes their removal from cells by repairing damaged "cleaning systems" in the neurons. As discussed in Part 1, the most common theory of Alzheimer's causation points to beta-amyloid and tau protein buildup. Scientists now speculate that inflammation develops to clear the plaques and tangles and damages surrounding tissue. As the disease progresses, massive cell loss withers and shrinks the brain.

> In addition to slowing beta-amyloid and tau protein production, lithium promotes their removal from cells by repairing damaged "cleaning systems" in the neurons.

Nerve cells regularly are broken down and removed. However, in patients with Alzheimer's disease and other neurodegenerative diseases, this process is disabled. This allows peptides and tau proteins to accumulate much faster in a more destructive manner.[15] In this process, waste is not disposed of properly. As in many body systems, a buildup of waste can devastate connected systems.

Lithium encourages the removal of unwanted nerve cell components by inhibiting the enzyme inositol monophosphatase (IMPase). Normally, IMPase promotes recycling of important signaling molecules in the cells.[16] When lithium blocks IMPase, this recycling stops, and any waste is cleared. It thereby corrects the waste removal process so that harmful proteins are eliminated without hurting healthy tissues.[17,18]

Lithium Helps Healthy Cells Survive

When cells are too damaged to be cleaned or repaired, they shrink, fall apart, and die. The process of apoptosis, or cell death, clears cells that have been overrun with misfolded proteins and can no longer function. In many patients with Alzheimer's, apoptosis goes awry, and cell death is triggered in random nervous system cells.[19] Lithium counteracts this effect by suppressing the molecules that initiate cell death. At the same time, lithium supports the expression of molecules that mark cells as healthy so they are not mistaken as needing apoptosis.[20-22] By recalibrating the rate of cell death in the nervous system, lithium has remarkable potential to stop the accelerated and unchecked tissue loss that accompanies Alzheimer's disease and other neurodegenerative illnesses.

> Lithium has remarkable potential to stop the accelerated and unchecked tissue loss that accompanies Alzheimer's disease and other neurodegenerativeillnesses.

Lithium Regulates Glutamate and Decreases Inflammation

Glutamate is the most important neurotransmitter for normal brain function. Over half of all brain synapses release glutamate in order to communicate. Under healthy conditions, glutamate promotes the biological processes involved with learning and memory. However, excess glutamate can overwhelm the neurons, leading to agitation, injury, and cell death.[23] This often occurs in the Alzheimer's brain, where too much excitatory glutamate floods cells.

Lithium prevents glutamate uptake into the cells by deactivating N-methyl-D-aspartate (NMDA) receptors, the main class of glutamate receptors in the nervous tissue. Balancing glutamate levels is another way that lithium may prevent cell death associated with Alzheimer's and related symptoms of cognitive decline. Remarkably, lithium exerts these effects when used at doses considered low by mainstream medicine.[24]

Neuroinflammation, or inflammation of nervous tissue, occurs normally as a protective process coordinated by the immune system in response to an infection or injury. It then stimulates repair and recovery by delivering white blood cells. However, if not controlled, this process can be very damaging. Lithium stabilizes this process and decreases inflammation in different ways.

> Scientists now believe that the inflammatory response becomes disrupted and proceeds in an out-of-control way in Alzheimer's disease.

Lithium suppresses pro-inflammatory cytokines. Scientists now believe that the inflammatory response becomes disrupted and proceeds in an out-of-control way in Alzheimer's disease.[25,26] Control over this process may help arrest neuron destruction and stabilize brain health. Cells in the immune system communicate by releasing and responding to chemical messengers such as cytokines. Lithium moderates inflammation by dampening cytokine reactivity. It also suppresses the immune cells in the brain and spinal cord, preventing them from overstimulation.[26]

Lithium treatment changes fatty acid metabolism in the brain to protect against inflammation. It does so by blocking the release of an unstable and reactive fatty acid and bolstering a fatty acid that helps repair cells.[27]

Lithium May Stabilize Calcium Ions and Can Influence Genes

Although calcium plays a vital role in cell health, excess calcium ions can damage cells. Too much calcium in a cell can even lead to cell death. Researcher James Wallace advanced the theory that calcium ions play a role in Alzheimer's disease.[28] Controlling calcium ions, then, might delay cognitive decline. Lithium has been shown to reduce calcium ion concentrations. Wallace hypothesized that lithium protects against cognitive decline by stabilizing calcium ions. Studies are underway to test this idea.

We now know that lithium can even change the way genes are expressed. Already, scientists have upended our former understanding of genetics. Ever since Gregor Mendel's research, genetic heritage was considered fixed at birth, in contrast to the idea that environmental forces influence individuals as they grow. "Nature" and "nurture" were thought of as opposing forces. We now realize that the influence of genetics on health is much more complicated than just the DNA sequence in our genes. We have a new understanding based on science: our genetic code is more changeable than we knew. Although genes themselves may not change, whether and how much a gene is expressed are infinitely variable.

> Lithium's dramatic effects on the brain go beyond changes at the cellular level. We now know that lithium can even change the way genes are expressed.

The exciting new field based on these discoveries is called *epigenetics*, the study of how people's environments and experiences affect their gene function. Epigenetic changes are long-lasting changes in gene function that do not change the genetic code. They form the link between environmental and genetic factors.[29-31] In contrast to the static DNA sequence, the epigenome, or the many chemical compounds surrounding the genome and directing its activity, can be changed. It is, in fact, quite responsive to the environment, our emotions, and our diet. The epigenome is like a light switch that turns on or off the expression of specific genes. Through the epigenome, environmental factors profoundly influence gene expression.

The chemical reason that genes do not determine health in a uniform way is that they carry chemical attachments that act on DNA to regulate the timing and amount of the gene without changing its basic composition. These chemical attachments, or epigenetic markers, determine whether a gene is expressed or silenced.

Lithium is a powerful epigenetic factor that can protect the brain in several ways. It changes gene expression by acting on DNA and the BDNF gene. By ensuring that the BDNF gene is left in the "on" position, lithium promotes consistent release of substances that protect and nourish the brain.[30]

> Lithium is a powerful epigenetic factor that can protect the brain in several ways.

BDNF levels are diminished in both the brain and the serum of patients with Alzheimer's disease. In one study, Alzheimer's patients treated for 10 weeks with lithium showed a significant increase in BDNF levels. They also had less cognitive impairment than a similar group of patients with Alzheimer's treated with placebo.[31]

Lithium also acts by changing the proteins called histones. Histone function is especially important for encoding functions like learning and memory. In fact, diminished memory in Alzheimer's patients has been linked with problems in the way the body uses histones. In laboratory animals, lithium made histones more available to proteins that enhance memory.[32]

Although studies in humans are needed to further explain how it works, lithium may prevent the genetic changes associated with Alzheimer's disease and similar conditions. The field of epigenetics is new, but we already know that lithium promotes genetic changes that affect the expression of more than 50 genes.[33] As research shows us how to manipulate gene expression and suppression, targeted use of lithium will help us better prevent and treat disorders that now lead to neurological decline.

Lithium helps nerve cells grow and survive. It modulates multiple biological cascades involved with nerve cell development and increases levels of key proteins involved in nerve cell development. Other studies have shown that lithium protects neurons by reducing inflammation, enhancing mitochondrial function, and increasing antioxidants. Imaging studies have even provided visual evidence that patients taking lithium salts experience increases in brain tissue over time, particularly in gray matter. At the cellular level, lithium exerts powerful influences on neuroprotection and brain health. Lithium, then, protects against changes associated with Alzheimer's disease through many pathways.

> Lithium helps nerve cells grow and survive.

Summary

Since lithium has been shown to protect cells from deterioration and even promote regeneration, scientific knowledge has grown about how lithium works in Alzheimer's disease. Lithium protects neurons and promotes growth of new neurons. This has exciting implications for the aging brain in that brain shrinkage and brain cell loss can be reversed.

In addition, lithium increases levels of NAA to enhance nerve cell metabolism. Lithium inhibits GSK3, slowing the production of plaques and tangles. It also stimulates the clearing of plaques and tangles. Lithium relieves the brain of excessive glutamate and its excitotoxic effects and reduces inflammation. Finally, through its effects on BDNF and histones, lithium may help prevent genetic changes linked to Alzheimer's disease.

Key Points

- Lithium has shown the ability to increase the volume of the hippocampus, the part of the brain most involved in memory.

- Lithium helps remove cell wastes, including plaques and tangles. It also helps prevent death of healthy cells.
- Lithium controls inflammation.
- Lithium contributes to genetic changes that diminish the severity of Alzheimer's disease.

10
LITHIUM'S BROADER BENEFITS
FOR LIFELONG BRAIN HEALTH

In a previous chapter, we focused on how lithium protects against Alzheimer's disease. Beyond these effects on Alzheimer's and other dementias, lithium contributes to brain health in other ways.

Lithium Balances Neurotransmitter Levels

Neurotransmitters are chemical messengers that help coordinate mood, appetite, sleep, movement, and other vital processes that support health. Sustaining an appropriate balance of these compounds is critical to our mental and physiological health.

Lithium enhances serotonin, a key neurotransmitter that contributes to feelings of well-being, satisfaction, and happiness. Studies in humans have shown that lithium optimizes the amount of serotonin available for use in the brain and other body systems.[1-3]

Animal studies have shown that lithium supports and balances the serotonergic system in several ways.[4] For example, lithium ions can repair problems with the synthesis, uptake, storage, and release of serotonin to ensure that an appropriate amount is available to the cells. Some studies have suggested that lithium improves the operation of serotonin receptors as well.[5] Therefore, lithium not only increases serotonin levels but also helps regulate its transport throughout the nervous system.

In addition, lithium modulates dopamine, a neurotransmitter that influences movement, emotion, and cognition. This neurotransmitter is most widely noted for its role in the brain's reward system. Positive experiences, tasty foods, and addictive drugs trigger a rush of dopamine, leading to better focus, motivation, and feelings of pleasure.

For this reward system to function properly, dopamine must be released in precise, well-timed amounts. If too much dopamine floods the cells, it can cause agitation. Lithium appears to counteract dopamine-induced hyperactivity and restore dopamine transport.[6,7] Conversely, lithium can increase dopamine activity when levels are too low. These complementary results reveal that the actions of lithium are not simple and one-directional. Instead, they depend on other factors as well as the condition of the brain.

> In addition, lithium modulates dopamine, a dynamic neurotransmitter that influences movement, emotion, and cognition.

Lithium Modulates Monoamine Oxidase Activity

Monoamine oxidase (MAO) is an enzyme that breaks down certain neurotransmitters in the body such as dopamine, and serotonin. Levels of MAO determine how much of a neurotransmitter is available to neurons at any time. In a healthy nervous system, MAO activity is highly regulated to maintain balanced neurotransmitter levels.

When MAO activity decreases, neurotransmitters are not broken down properly, and too much can remain in the nervous system. This imbalance often occurs in cases of chronic aggression and the manic phase of bipolar disorder, in which elevated dopamine and norepinephrine drive impulsive, sensation-seeking behaviors. Lower MAO activity has been associated with greater severity and frequency of impulsive, violent, or abusive behaviors as well.[8]

In these circumstances, lithium stabilizes MAO activity by increasing its ability to break down excitatory neurotransmitters.[9] Interestingly, evidence also shows that lithium can reduce MAO activity,[9] which would prove useful in conditions like depression, in which lower neurotransmitter levels may be the key issue. The complementary actions suggest that lithium has adaptogenic effects on the MAO system. Lithium appears to calibrate enzyme activity in either direction, depending on what is needed to achieve homeostasis.

Lithium Provides Metabolic Support

The mineral lithium is absorbed through the small intestine. It is then distributed throughout the body and deposited in bone and hair.[10] Along the way, lithium ions interact with other nutrients to carry out several important tasks.

Lithium is needed to transport vitamin B12 and folate into cells.[10] These vitamins affect the central nervous system and work together to support processes that stabilize behavior and cognitive function. Lithium helps support healthy intercellular communication in the nervous system by helping vitamin B12 and folate move across cell membranes. This is a basic pathway through which lithium regulates mood and behavior.[10]

Oxidative stress occurs when there are too many damaging molecules known as free radicals for the body to counteract with antioxidants. Free radicals regularly and negatively alter fats, proteins, and DNA that constitute brain cells, causing diseases in the nervous system. Researchers think that cumulative, long-term exposure to free radicals in the environment damages cells.

Lithium curbs free radicals by increasing antioxidant defenses in the nervous system.[11] Primarily, it increases levels of glutathione in the brain.[12] Glutathione is an antioxidant found naturally in every cell in the body. While many vitamins, minerals, and phytochemicals also act as antioxidants, glutathione is

> Lithium curbs free radicals by increasing antioxidant defenses in the peripheral and central nervous systems.

unique because it is made in the cell. Adequate glutathione levels are required for antioxidants to be effectively used. By boosting production of glutathione, the "master antioxidant," lithium protects the nervous system by reinforcing the entire antioxidant network in cells.

Lithium Improves Mitochondrial Function

Most diseases of the brain involve a reduction in neuron metabolism, often due to a malfunction in the mitochondria—the organelles that generate energy for cells. As the powerhouses of the cell, mitochondria are part of a broad range of basic functions and are vital to the maintenance of healthy cells and tissues.

Mitochondrial defects are found in a striking number of health conditions, including Alzheimer's disease and aging. Recognition of this connection has made the mitochondria a focus of development of early detection and treatment strategies.[13]

Lithium improves mitochondrial function by increasing mitochondrial mass and their ability to generate energy for cells.[14,15] For dementia sufferers, the mitochondrial support of lithium can help re-ignite failing brain tissue metabolism.

> For dementia sufferers, the mitochondrial support of lithium can help re-ignite failing brain tissue metabolism.

Summary

Lithium contributes to brain health in broad ways. It balances neurotransmitter levels and modulates MAO activity. Lithium interacts with other nutrients to perform critical metabolic functions. By increasing antioxidant defenses in the nervous system, lithium protects against free radicals.

Key Points

- Lithium enhances serotonin available in the brain and other body systems.
- Lithium regulates MAO, maintaining balanced neurotransmitter levels.
- Lithium facilitates vitamin B12 and folate transfer across cell membranes.
- By curbing free radicals, lithium protects against oxidative stress.
- Lithium increases mitochondrial mass, generating more cell energy.

11
THE FASCINATING HISTORY OF ELEMENT 3: WATER AND TECHNOLOGY

Lithium wields its molecular magic by preventing brain changes related to Alzheimer's disease and protecting brain health throughout life. Before you make lithium a part of your own diet (as is discussed in the following chapter), you may find it interesting to learn about the history of this amazing mineral in water and medicine and its current applications in technology.

Even the soft drink entrepreneur Charles Leiper Grigg understood there was something special about the naturally occurring element lithium. In 1929, he unveiled a soft drink called Bib-Label Lithiated Lemon-Lime Soda with the slogan, "It takes the ouch out of the grouch." Hailed for improving mood and curing hangovers, this product was eventually rechristened 7-Up. The "7" supposedly represents the rounded-up atomic weight of the element lithium (6.9), and the "Up" suggests its power to lift spirits. Lithium remained an ingredient of 7-Up until 1950.[1]

Centuries before the advent of this celebrated soft drink, lithium was associated with calming moods. Soranus, a physician from ancient Ephesus, observed the benefits of alkaline springs for soothing the wild spirits of some of his patients. Lithium, it turned out, was abundant in these springs.[2]

> The history of lithium has followed an amazing trajectory, from the calming springs of ancient Ephesus to the sophisticated technology of the space age.

Natural springs containing lithium were popular in both the eastern and the western hemispheres thought the 19th century. Archaeology has unearthed evidence that the mineral pools of what is now known as Lithia Springs, GA were a sacred site to indigenous peoples in the area. It remains a respected area for medicinal healing, and in 1890, the Lithia Springs Sanitarium was established to treat compulsive behaviors, including alcoholism and opioid dependence.[2]

The simple element lithium, which is plentiful in alkaline springs, gets its name from the Greek word for stone, *lithos*. Lithium is unevenly distributed on the earth. In addition to its presence in natural springs, lithium is found in granite and other rocks as well as in sea water. When rocks break down, lithium leaches into the soil, where it is readily absorbed by plants and enters the food chain. The most common source of lithium in the modern diet is tap water.[3]

Tap water contains calcium, magnesium, and sodium. It may also contain fluoride, added by the municipality to improve dental health. Tap water also contains trace minerals, which vary by geographical region.

The everyday water we drink comes from two sources: surface water and groundwater. Surface water is precipitation that falls from the sky in the form of rain or snow that collects in creeks, streams, rivers, ponds, and lakes. Groundwater is precipitation that seeps slowly into the soil and makes its way over time to deep underground aquifers. When rain or snow falls, it contains no minerals other than material it picks up on the way down. Water absorbs minerals from its contact with the earth. Surface water, because of its limited contact with the ground, has a lower concentration of minerals than groundwater. Local geology determines which minerals leach into the water. In the Midwest, for example, where the ground contains limestone, groundwater picks up calcium and magnesium. In the Northwest, where there are deposits of granite and basalt, water picks up iron and manganese. Because of geographical variation, groundwater may have high concentrations of some important minerals but be entirely devoid of others. Water can also absorb minerals that are harmful in any dose, including lead, arsenic, and industrial pollutants. It is not uncommon to find trace amounts of lithium in the water supply. And its effect on the population that drinks it is positive.

Two researchers made an amazing discovery in 1990, and we are still realizing its exciting implications.[4] They conducted a large study based on the realization that naturally occurring levels of trace lithium in municipal water supplies vary from county to county. The drinking water in some counties contains no lithium, while trace amounts are present in other counties. The researchers' analysis of data from 27 counties from 1978 to 1987 showed that the incidence rates of suicide, homicide, and rape were significantly higher in counties where the water supply contained little or no lithium in contrast to counties with water lithium levels ranging from 70 to 170 micrograms per liter. Incidence rates of robbery, burglary, and theft showed the same statistically significant pattern.[4]

> The researchers' analysis of data from 27 counties from 1978 to 1987 showed that the incidence rates of suicide, homicide, and rape were significantly higher in counties where the water supply contained little or no lithium.

Further comparisons of drinking water lithium levels with incidents of arrests for possession of opium, cocaine, and their derivatives also revealed statistically significant inverse relationships. The researchers concluded their study by suggesting that supplementation, or lithiation, of drinking water could effectively reduce crime, suicide, and drug dependency at the individual and community levels.

There is increasing evidence that trace amounts of lithium in municipal water supplies lower suicide rates among those served by the water system. Several studies in different countries have analyzed data about suicide incidence and the presence or absence of lithium in the water supply. A Japanese study analyzed data from 18 municipalities with more than one million inhabitants over five years.[5] The Japanese researchers confirmed the findings of the earlier study: suicide and crime rates were inversely correlated with the lithium content in the local water supply. Lithium levels were significantly and inversely related to the suicide mortality ratio for each municipality.[5]

A more recent study in Japan evaluated the association between lithium levels in tap water and suicide in 40 municipalities of Aomori prefecture, which has the highest rates of suicide in Japan.[6] Studies in Greece and Austria have corroborated these results. These studies suggest the potential power of lithium as a supplement to improve nutritional health.

Lithium in Manufacturing and Technology

No overview of lithium's uses would be complete without acknowledging the element's importance to the world of manufacturing and technology. Only about 5% of the world's lithium supply is actually used for health-related purposes. The remaining 95% is used in industry.

Lithium is extracted from the earth using two different methods: mining lithium ores and mining lithium brines in salt lakes. Beginning in the late 1990s, brines became the main source because processing hard rock ore is more expensive. Brine deposits, which represent about 66% of the global lithium supply, are found mainly in the salt flats of Chile, Argentina, China, and Tibet. There is only one brine operation in the United States.[7]

Recent high demand for lithium in industry has led to increased mining and production. Lithium's properties ensure many uses in technology. The lightest of all solid elements, lithium is strong yet highly reactive, malleable, and a good conductor of heat and electricity. For many years, lithium compounds have been used to make ceramic, glass, and aluminum products. Because of lithium, Corning and Pyrex cookware, for instance, can be moved from refrigerator to oven without shattering. Lithium helps decrease thermal expansion and increase shock resistance.[8]

Lithium in varied forms has a broad range of applications. It is responsible for the color red in fireworks displays. As a metal, lithium is commonly used for aircraft parts because it is light. Lithium is in greatest demand for use in batteries. Its advantages include low weight and high energy density and electric output. Lithium batteries have become popular in aerospace because they are virtually maintenance free. The Mars Rovers used lithium batteries. For Spirit and Opportunity, the batteries successfully supported the entry, descent, landing, and post-landing operations.[9] Lithium has also drawn the attention of automotive manufacturers in their quest to develop environmentally friendly vehicles. Toyota, Honda, Nissan, Ford, Tesla, and other companies have produced successful prototype cars using lithium batteries. As battery production increases, costs decrease. Now the more than 59 lithium battery businesses in the United States bring in more than $3 billion in annual revenue.

The history of lithium has followed an amazing trajectory: from the calming springs of ancient Ephesus to the sophisticated technology of the space age. Lithium is revolutionizing aspects of technology, from batteries to automobiles, airplanes to space vehicles. Demand for lithium is on the rise because of its versatility, light weight, conductivity, high energy density, and malleability. Some economists predict that the lithium supply will soon drive the economy. This shape-shifting element clearly has a future even beyond its life-changing applications for health and disease.

Summary

Municipal tap water contains many trace minerals, which vary according to the geographical region and the minerals in the earth surrounding it. Groundwater is precipitation that seeps slowly through the soil and into deep underground aquifers. As it does, it absorbs minerals from the earth. In some areas, these natural minerals include lithium. Bottled distilled water is the only water with zero minerals.

A groundbreaking analysis of the drinking water in 27 Texas counties revealed that the incidence rates of theft and violent crime were significantly lower in the counties with drinking water that contained lithium. A Japanese study confirmed the Texas study's finding that suicide rates were lower when the lithium content in the local water supply was slightly higher.

Key Points

- Municipal tap water often contains calcium, magnesium, sodium, fluoride, and other trace minerals, which may include lithium. Bottled water may also contain minerals.
- In areas like the Midwest, where the ground contains limestone, groundwater picks up calcium and magnesium. In areas like the Northwest, where there's underlying granite and basalt, the water picks up iron and manganese.
- In May 1990, G.N. Schrauzer and K.P. Shrestha published their groundbreaking Texas research paper. Their results "suggested that lithium has moderating effects on suicidal and violent criminal behavior at levels that may be encountered in municipal water supplies."
- Lithium is a versatile mineral used in everything from cookware to aircraft, and demand is on the rise.

12
HOW TO MAKE LITHIUM PART OF YOUR DIET

Based on the overwhelming evidence that low-dose nutritional lithium can improve brain health and even turn back cognitive decline, the question becomes: How can I make this mineral a part of my diet? Fortunately, you can derive the positive effects of lithium even if it is not part of your local water supply.

Lithium in Nature

Unlike elements such as aluminum, carbon, gold, lead, silver, and tin, which occur naturally in the earth, lithium does not occur freely in nature. It is found only in compounds like pegmatitic minerals, igneous rocks composed almost entirely of crystals.

Because it is soluble as an ion, lithium is commonly found in brine, or water saturated with salt, from which most commercial lithium is harvested today. Brines are found underground, in salt lakes, or in seawater, or beneath the surface of lake beds. To extract lithium from brines, the salt-rich waters are pumped to the surface into evaporation ponds, where evaporation from the sun occurs over a number of months. Potassium is the first mineral to be harvested, and as the water evaporates, the ponds contain increasingly high concentrations of lithium. When lithium chloride in the ponds reaches an optimal concentration, the solution is pumped to a recovery plant, where extraction and filtering remove any unwanted material.

Lithium in Foods

Because lithium is found in soil and water, used in growing plants and raising livestock, trace lithium can be found in both vegetarian and non-vegetarian diets.

Seafood and Meats. Lithium from seawater concentrates in crustaceans and mollusks, including shrimp, lobster, oysters, and scallops. Lithium is present to a very small extent in fish. Dairy, eggs, and meat also contain slight concentrations of the trace mineral. Dairy products, including milk and cheese, are a significant natural source of lithium. Since lithium is a salt, it is absorbed from food and water by dairy cattle and released into milk.

> Because lithium is found in soil and water and used both in growing plants and raising livestock, trace lithium can be found in both vegetarian and non-vegetarian diets.

Legumes. Legumes, including dried peas and beans, lentils, chickpeas, and soybeans, contain some of the highest amounts of lithium available in food.

Vegetables. Although they contain less lithium than legumes, most vegetables contain some lithium because they absorb it from the soil. The highest lithium content is in the nightshade vegetables: potatoes, peppers, and tomatoes. The sea vegetable kelp, blue corn, and mustard from fresh mustard seeds contain trace amounts of lithium.

Grains and Nuts. Dried fruits and seeds contain miniscule amounts of lithium. Grains, especially wheat and rice products, have some lithium content. Coffee and pistachios are a known source of trace lithium.

Lithium Supplements

To realize the neuroprotective benefits of lithium, I recommend taking a supplement in addition to deriving trace amounts of lithium from food.

Low doses of lithium salts, a fraction of the pharmacological dose, can be purchased without prescription in health food stores across the United States. While regulations for sale of nutritional lithium vary widely around the world, lithium supplements are recognized as a dietary food by the FDA. Lithium supplements are generally prepared and dispensed as capsules, tablets, or liquid solutions. They are also available in different preparations, as lithium must be compounded with a mineral carrier in order for the body to safely absorb it.

> To realize the neuroprotective benefits of lithium, I recommend taking a supplement—either lithium orotate or lithium citrate—in addition to deriving trace lithium from food.

Nutritional lithium is intended to supplement the diet and does not require routine blood tests to establish a therapeutic level. Many patients can benefit from low doses without concerns about adverse side effects or toxicity.

Lithium aspartate and lithium orotate are available as capsules, and lithium citrate and lithium chloride are available as liquid solutions for purchase without a doctor's prescription. I recommend lithium orotate or lithium citrate for nutritional supplementation. Aspartate belongs to a class of chemicals called excitotoxins, which cause neurons to transmit impulses at such a rapid rate that receptors quickly become exhausted. The overstimulation can cause problems such as headaches and, possibly, inflammation. Studies that have compared lithium orotate to lithium carbonate have found that lower

> Studies that have compared lithium orotate to lithium carbonate have found that lower doses of lithium orotate can achieve therapeutic brain lithium concentrations while avoiding toxicity.

doses of lithium orotate can achieve therapeutic brain lithium concentrations while avoiding toxicity.[1]

Testing for Individual Lithium Need

In 1985, the U.S. Environmental Protection Agency estimated that Americans consume from 0.6 to 3.1 milligrams of lithium a day through water, vegetables, and grains.[2] To determine whether a patient has a lithium deficiency, I examine the results of a hair tissue mineral analysis. This simple, inexpensive, and noninvasive procedure can evaluate long-term patterns of lithium storage in the body. Hair testing can be done from the comfort of home and does not require any special laboratory equipment or handling instructions.

Hair Tissue Mineral Analysis: Using a clean pair of scissors, small amounts of hair are collected from five different locations on the scalp, close to the scalp and including the back of the head. A small amount of the collected hair is submitted to a lab through regular postal mail. The analysis takes about three or four weeks. The laboratory assesses levels and ratios of minerals, including lithium, zinc, copper, and magnesium, as well as levels of toxic chemicals such as arsenic, lead, and mercury.

Hair analysis is a reliable indicator of lithium deficiency because hair is one of the many places where the body eliminates minerals and metals. Hair analyses reflect the status of bioavailable lithium for, on average, two or three months before rather than the snapshot image blood plasma offers.[3] The individual mineral levels, ratios, and patterns of minerals deposited in the hair can reveal how well the body is functioning at a cellular level.[4] Moreover, lithium levels are higher in hair than blood, making it easier to detect and measure in the hair.[5] Blood tests of lithium can be unreliable in detecting a physiological deficiency.

> A hair analysis is a reliable indicator of lithium deficiency because hair is one of the many places where the body eliminates minerals and metals.

The procedure for preparing and analyzing samples is provided in the hair sample collection kit, which provides step-by-step instructions, ensuring uniformity in collection techniques. Since 1975, researchers have published data on lithium levels in the human body based on lithium levels obtained through hair analysis. Data from many populations around the world are now available for comparison. The results from a hair tissue mineral analysis can offer tremendous insight about the likely benefit of low-dose lithium therapy.

Urine Test. Another option is the recently developed urine test. Lithium is almost completely absorbed through the gastrointestinal tract, with the kidney serving as the main pathway for lithium elimination from the body. Most ingested lithium is excreted in urine within 24 hours, making it a good indicator for total lithium passage through the body from recent dietary intake.

> Most ingested lithium is excreted in urine within 24 hours, making it a good indicator for total lithium passage through the body from recent dietary intake.

ZRT Laboratory in Beaverton, OR has developed a test for measuring lithium levels using dried urine as the sample type. This allows stable preservation of the sample and ensures ease of collection and shipping. The lab compares the individual sample result with a reference range for lithium established based on levels determined from a healthy patient population.

Dosage Recommendations. I recommend supplementation with lithium orotate. For individuals older than 40, a suggested dose is 2.5 mg per day to counteract the cognitive decline associated with the aging process. For patients who already have symptoms of cognitive decline, I recommend dose ranges of 5 to 10 mg of lithium orotate.

Before initiating low-dose lithium, screen for thyroid disorders. Like any other nutritional mineral such as iron or calcium, lithium can be toxic in high doses. If you have symptoms of lithium toxicity, such as nausea, vomiting, diarrhea, drowsiness, muscle weakness, tremor, lack of coordination, blurred vision, or ringing in your ears, stop taking lithium and talk with your doctor. I have been prescribing nutritional lithium for 30 years and have observed no adverse effects during that time.

Summary

Supplementing your diet with a nutritional dose of lithium can protect your brain in the many ways discussed in previous chapters. Even if trace lithium is not part of your local water supply, you can drive the benefits of lithium through your diet and supplementation. Lithium levels are tested through a simple, noninvasive procedure, the hair tissue mineral analysis.

I recommend an initial dose of 2.5 to 5 mg per day of lithium orotate. If you have symptoms of cognitive decline, the initial dose should be 5 to 10 mg. If you take lithium, you should be monitored by a health professional. During more than 30 years of prescribing nutritional lithium, I have witnessed no adverse effects except for rare complaints of feeling "too calm."

Key Points

- Trace amounts of lithium are found in a variety of foods, including seafood and meats, legumes, vegetables, grains, and nuts.
- A low dose of a nutritional supplement can protect against cognitive decline.
- Low doses of lithium are recommended, as they have greater efficacy for cognitive symptoms, and high doses can be toxic.
- People taking lithium should be monitored by a health professional.

Step-by-Step Action Plan for Preventing Alzheimer's Disease with Low-Dose Lithium

Step #1: To determine if you are deficient in lithium, order a hair tissue mineral analysis kit from Great Plains Laboratory (greatplainslaboratory.com) or a urine test from ZRT Laboratory (zrtlab.com).*

Step #2: Start lithium supplementation:

- Lithium orotate, 2.5 mg/day, or liquid lithium citrate, 1.0 mg/day
- Luma (JayMac Pharmaceuticals) – A multinutrient Alzheimer's prevention supplement with 2.5 mg of lithium orotate per tablet (lumaforlife.com)

Liquid lithium (Pure Encapsulations) – A liquid preparation of lithium citrate, 2 mg (pureencapsulations.com)

*Lithium Deficiency is not recognized by the Food and Nutrition Board of the Institute of Medicine in the National Academy of Sciences.

Warning: Lithium should not be taken by pregnant or lactating women. Low-dose lithium is not a replacement for prescription lithium for patients with bipolar disorder. Do not take lithium if you have thyroid or kidney disease. Do not exceed 5.0 mg a day of lithium without being monitored by a health professional.

PART 4
NUTRITIONAL SUPPORT FOR ALZHEIMER'S PREVENTION

13
THE DANGERS OF HOMOCYSTEINE
AND HOW TO MEASURE IT

By now you see clearly that any supplements you take must be chosen wisely, and for good reason: not all supplements are made equally, nor are they equally effective at targeting the causes of aging, dementia, and Alzheimer's disease. In the following section of this book, I discuss supplements that clinical studies have shown help prevent the damaging effects of Alzheimer's.

To begin, let me explain the danger of a substance present at high levels in the blood of patients with Alzheimer's disease: homocysteine. Homocysteine is an amino acid in the blood. As people age, some brain atrophy, or loss of neurons, is common. But atrophy progresses faster in people with mild cognitive impairment and at a still faster rate in people with Alzheimer's disease. A factor that appears to accelerate brain atrophy and thereby double the risk of Alzheimer's is a high level of homocysteine in the blood. Homocysteine is made from another amino acid, methionine. It is normally converted into other amino acids for use by the body through a process called methylation, which sparks the activity of the body's cardiovascular, neurological, reproductive, and

A factor that appears to accelerate brain atrophy and thereby double the risk of Alzheimer's is a high level of homocysteine in the blood.

detoxification systems. Methylation of homocysteine allows the body to produce proteins and other essential compounds.

However, homocysteine that builds up unused in the body leads to a host of problems. Scientists have known for some time that elevated levels of this amino acid are associated with cardiovascular disease and stroke. Many studies have now shown that raised homocysteine concentrations in the blood also contribute to declining memory, poor judgment, and Alzheimer's disease.

A possible link between high levels of homocysteine and cognitive impairment was noted by investigators at Boston University and Tufts University in 2002.[1] To investigate this link, the research groups tested homocysteine levels in the blood of newly diagnosed Alzheimer's patients and compared them to the blood levels of subjects without symptoms of cognitive decline in the large, population-based Framingham Heart Study.[2] This long-term, ongoing cardiovascular study of residents of Framingham, MA began in 1946 and is now focused on its third generation of participants. The longitudinal nature of the study allowed the researchers to examine homocysteine levels in younger people without memory problems over years, well before symptoms of dementia developed. From 1986 to 1990, blood plasma homocysteine levels were measured in 1,092 participants considered "dementia-free." These participants, whose age was, on average, 76, had been enrolled in the study from 1976 to 1978. Plasma homocysteine was measured from 1979 to 1982 and from 1986 to 1990. Researchers also considered age, sex, and genetic risk factors.

From 1986 to 2000, some 111 people from the study developed dementia, including 83 diagnosed with Alzheimer's.[1] Elevated homocysteine levels doubled the chance that a participant would develop Alzheimer's disease, and each increment of elevation in level increased the risk of Alzheimer's by 40%. Participants with consistently high

> Independently, several research teams in different countries have documented a strong connection between high homocysteine levels and significantly increased Alzheimer's risk.

levels of homocysteine throughout the study period were at greatest risk for dementia and Alzheimer's disease. The researchers also examined whether homocysteine levels measured from 1979 to 1982 were related to developing Alzheimer's disease later in life. This analysis linked elevated levels of homocysteine at least eight years before to subsequent diagnosis of Alzheimer's disease. Researchers found the association between Alzheimer's disease and homocysteine both strong and independent of other factors, including age, sex, genotype, and other known and suspected risk factors.[1]

Research in Australia confirmed this strong association.[3] A total of 4,227 men 70 to 89 years old were examined to assess a possible link between homocysteine and Alzheimer's disease. The research team concluded that homocysteine accelerates the risk of Alzheimer's in older men; this risk increased by 48% when homocysteine concentrations were doubled. Analysis demonstrated that the link was independent of risk factors commonly associated with dementia, including age, education, smoking, alcohol, and vascular conditions.[3] The same research team found that high homocysteine in the blood was linked to lower performance on tests of memory retrieval and overall cognitive performance.

> The research team concluded that homocysteine accelerates the risk of Alzheimer's in older men; this risk increased by 48% when homocysteine concentrations were doubled.

Until 2009, exploration of a link between homocysteine levels and Alzheimer's disease had focused mostly on elderly men. A study in that year turned the spotlight on women and their homocysteine levels at midlife.[4] The investigators used data from the Prospective Population Study of Women in Gothenburg, Sweden begun in 1968.[5] This study had already enrolled large groups of women born in 1908, 1914, 1918, 1922, and 1930. Baseline homocysteine blood levels were available for 1,368 of the women. As the sample population reached ages when dementia is common, the researchers evaluated the women's cognitive functioning.

The study concluded that women with higher homocysteine levels earlier in life were most likely to develop Alzheimer's disease. They reached this conclusion by analyzing patterns of disease in women followed for 35 years. The research team speculated that homocysteine is directly related to processes that go wrong in the brain with Alzheimer's disease: stimulation of beta-amyloid production, a decrease in cholinesterases, activation of glutamate receptors, tau phosphorylation, and oxidative stress.[4]

Elevated homocysteine levels appear to be present in many diseases and conditions that afflict the elderly: Alzheimer's and other dementias, cardiovascular issues, stroke, and bone fracture. The researchers who worked with data from the Framingham Heart Study data speculate that these multiple connections point to the possibility of a common denominator or a single factor that may contribute significantly to all of these diseases. Whether the common denominator is homocysteine itself or whether high homocysteine is a marker for a still hidden condition is a pressing question for future research.[6]

Independently, several research teams in different countries have documented a strong connection between high homocysteine levels and a significantly increased risk of Alzheimer's disease. Scientists are excited to pinpoint this definitive link between an amino acid level in the blood and the process of cell degeneration and atrophy because it points to a way to intervene in this destructive process. The best part of this discovery is that a high homocysteine level, unlike genetic heritage, is changeable.

> Independently, several research teams in different countries have documented a strong connection between high homocysteine levels and a significantly increased risk of Alzheimer's disease.

The condition called hyperhomocysteinemia, or a high homocysteine level, can be diagnosed with a simple blood test, which I recommend. If your homocysteine level is high, take immediate steps to change it to reduce your risk of developing Alzheimer's disease. Fortunately, homocysteine levels are easily lowered through supplementation with the simple substances folic acid and other B vitamins. We explore these options in the following chapter.

Summary

Several large research studies have linked a history of high homocysteine levels with subsequent cognitive decline. Research has confirmed a connection between high homocysteine and the development of Alzheimer's disease in both men and women. A strong association between elevated homocysteine and Alzheimer's disease has been confirmed by a considerable body of research. Conclusive evidence of this link makes lowering homocysteine levels an urgent priority.

Key Points

- High levels of homocysteine can double the risk of Alzheimer's disease.
- The link between earlier homocysteine levels and later Alzheimer's has been confirmed by analyses of large studies of men and women, the Framingham Heart Study and the prospective population study of women in Gothenburg.
- Homocysteine levels can be measured by a simple blood test.

14
FOLIC ACID AND OTHER B VITAMINS LOWER HOMOCYSTEINE

Because research studies associate high homocysteine and Alzheimer's disease, lowering homocysteine levels should be a high priority. Homocysteine builds up in the blood when metabolism is impaired. This impairment often results from a lack of B vitamins, particularly folic acid, B6, and B12. Luckily, these deficiencies can be tested for and supplemented.

> Because research studies associate high homocysteine and Alzheimer's disease, lowering homocysteine levels should be a high priority.

Folic acid, or vitamin B9, has strong neuroprotective properties. After scientists discovered decades ago that it is effective in preventing neural tube defects in babies, fortification of wheat flour with folic acid is now mandatory in the United States, Australia, Canada, and several other countries.

Folic acid is required for normal cell development and the manufacture of DNA and RNA. It has also been shown in multiple research studies to reduce homocysteine levels in the blood.

The Difference Between Folate, Folic acid, and L-methylfolate

First, a clarification of terms: although these terms are sometimes used interchangeably, they are different forms of the same vitamin. As a result, the body handles them differently. This is important to recognize when determining which supplements are most needed.

- Folate is the natural form of vitamin B9 present in various foods.
- Folic acid is the manmade form of the vitamin B9 used in supplements and fortified foods. This is the form people usually take as a supplement. It directly affects metabolism in the body but not in the brain.
- 5-methyltetrahydrofolate (also known as L-methylfolate or 5-MTHF) is the natural form of folate used at the cellular level for DNA reproduction and regulation of homocysteine.

L-methylfolate easily crosses the blood-brain barrier, the system of specialized capillaries that regulates compounds entering the brain. The capillaries constituting the blood-brain barrier serve the entire central nervous system, allowing certain substances to cross it while fencing others out. In order to affect the brain and influence mental well-being, folate must first be changed into L-methylfolate so that it can cross this barrier. After entering the brain, this form of folate helps create and maintain neurotransmitters.

MTHFR Mutation. Many people's bodies easily and efficiently change the folate they get from food and folic acid from supplements into the active forms needed for optimal body and brain function. But others do not due to their genetics. MTHF is an enzyme needed for methylation, the process by which folic acid is converted into an active form the body can use. The MTHFR gene produces this enzyme, but a genetic

An estimated 30% of the population has the MTHFR mutation, which means that a third of the population cannot process folate or folic acid on their own and convert them into their active form.

mutation can inhibit its function. An estimated 30% of the population has the MTHFR mutation, which means that a third of the population cannot process folate or folic acid on their own and convert them into their active form, L-methylfolate. Not surprisingly, those with this mutation can eat plenty of folate-containing foods and take folate supplements, but the amount of folate that reaches the brain is low. Therefore, these nutrients area unable to carry out one of their key functions: breaking down homocysteine. For this reason, people with a MTHFR mutation often have high levels of homocysteine.

Testing for Folate and the MTHFR Mutation

No single test determines whether you have enough folate, as folate levels in the blood do not always accurately reflect the folate levels in the area surrounding the brain. Another way to indirectly measure folate in the brain is to check for homocysteine levels as listed in the previous chapter, since folate is responsible for reducing homocysteine levels in the blood.

Since an estimated 30% of the population has the MTHFR mutation, I recommend both taking a MTHFR genetic test and folic acid supplementation in the form of L-methylfolate. Many companies offer this test as a noninvasive saliva swab, so you just need to send it back and wait for your results. L-methylfolate supplements (as opposed to folate, folic acid, or vitamin B9 supplements) can be purchased over the counter in some pharmacies, vitamin stores, and health food stores. In addition, folate in this form has fewer health risks than commonly used synthetic folic acid supplements. I suggest a minimum dose of 3 to 5 mg of L-methylfolate a day to protect against memory loss and Alzheimer's disease.

> I recommend both taking a MTHFR genetic test and folic acid supplementation in the form of L-methylfolate.

Vitamins B6 and B12

In addition to folic acid, or vitamin B9, considerable research echoes the findings that taking vitamins B6 and B12 also significantly lowers homocysteine levels. A meta-analysis, or large evaluation of many research studies, concluded that daily doses of these B vitamins reduce homocysteine levels to 31% of their previous level.[1] Because this analysis was based on results from many studies, the researchers were confident in concluding that a daily dose of B vitamins can reduce an individual's homocysteine levels by a third.[1] Boosting your intake of folate, vitamin B6, and vitamin B12 will help return homocysteine levels to normal. A safe, simple, and inexpensive treatment with B vitamins, then, slows the rate of brain atrophy.

How to Lower Homocysteine with Diet, Vitamin B, and Lifestyle

Diet also is an opportunity to lower homocysteine levels by increasing levels of B vitamins. To consume more **folate**, eat:
- Leafy green vegetables such as spinach
- Many breakfast cereals and other fortified grain products
- Most types of beans
- Lentils
- Asparagus

> Diet also is an opportunity to lower homocysteine levels by increasing levels of B vitamins.

Foods rich in **vitamin B6** include:
- Fortified breakfast cereals
- Bananas
- Garbanzo beans (chickpeas)
- Potatoes
- Chicken

Good sources of **vitamin B12** include:

- Beef
- Dairy products (keep in mind, however, that high levels of homocysteine may be associated with an excess of red meat and dairy.)
- Organ meats (such as liver)
- Some types of fish

While taking vitamin B supplements to lower homocysteine, you may want to consider making other **lifestyle changes** to that may address possible causes of high homocysteine as well:

> Supplements to correct any metabolic imbalances resulting in high levels of homocysteine must be taken with consideration of their relative levels and your ability to absorb them.

- Examining your prescription drug use. Some, including cholestyramine, colestipol, fenofibrate, levodopa, metformin, methotrexate, niacin, nitrous oxide, pemetrexed, phenytoin, and sulfasalazine, may be associated with higher levels of homocysteine.
- Cutting down on smoking, coffee, and alcohol.
- Exercising daily (patients in cardiac rehabilitation programs have reduced their homocysteine levels by exercise alone).

Few adverse effects from vitamin B have been observed at the low doses required to reduce homocysteine levels. Although vitamin B6 is water soluble and excreted in the urine, long-term supplementation with very high doses (over 200 mg) is not recommended and may result in symptoms known as sensory neuropathy. No toxic or adverse effects

> No toxic or adverse effects have been associated with vitamin B12 from food or supplements in healthy people.

have been associated with vitamin B12 from food or supplements in healthy people. Oral folic acid is generally nontoxic but may cause neurological injury in patients with undiagnosed pernicious anemia and may affect seizure control in patients with epilepsy. If this is a risk for you, please take this into consideration.

Summary

The neuroprotective properties of folic acid, or vitamin B9, were identified decades ago. Because it effectively prevents neural tube defects, folic acid fortification of wheat flour is now mandatory in several countries, including the United States.

Folic acid reduces homocysteine levels in blood. A study in the Netherlands showed that folate not only lowers homocysteine but also diminishes symptoms of cognitive decline. Other studies have demonstrated with MRI scans a visible reduction in brain atrophy in people taking folate.

Vitamin B6 and B12 yield positive effects on homocysteine levels beyond the effects of folate alone. Large studies have concluded that a daily dose of B vitamins can lower homocysteine levels by a third. Vitamin B supplements are a safe and inexpensive intervention to help protect your brain against Alzheimer's disease.

Key Points

- Folic acid reduces homocysteine levels in blood.
- This vitamin occurs in several forms: folic acid, folate, and L-methylfolate, the natural form of folate that crosses the blood-brain barrier.
- In people with the MTHFR mutation, folate is not converted to the active form. Taking L-methylfolate can bypass this potential problem.
- The B vitamins are also present in various foods. A combination of a diet rich in vitamin B, exercise, and vitamin B supplementation can stop the damage caused by dangerous homocysteine levels.

Step-by-Step Action Plan for Lowering Homocysteine Levels

Step #1: Ask your doctor to order blood tests for vitamin B12, folate, and a genetic test, usually a cheek swab for the MTHFR gene.

Step #2: If your doctor tells you that you have elevated homocysteine levels (more than 11 μmol/L), you must determine if the low level is related to B12 deficiency or folate deficiency.

Step #3: If deficient in vitamin B12 (blood test values are less than 500 ng/mL), take at least 5,000 mcg of methylcobalamin daily. If your level is less than 400 ng/mL, talk with your doctor about vitamin B12 injections.

Step #4: If you have any of the genetic variants on the MTHFR gene, take L-methylfolate 1-5 mg/day.

Step #5: There are nutritional supplements that combine all the nutrients that lower homocysteine, folate, vitamin B6, and vitamin B12.
- Luma (JayMac Pharmaceuticals) – A multinutrient Alzheimer's prevention supplement with 2.5 mg of lithium orotate per tablet (lumaforlife.com)

15
VITAMIN D AND ALZHEIMER'S

Vitamin D has many roles in maintaining health. It helps the body absorb calcium to build and maintain strong bones. It also helps muscles move, nerves carry messages between the brain and the rest of the body, and the immune system fight off bacteria and viruses. But what might surprise you is that vitamin D is involved in many of the processes of aging.

In humans, the most important compounds in the vitamin D group are vitamin D3 (cholecalciferol) and vitamin D2 (ergocalciferol). Both can be ingested from the diet and supplements. However, the major natural source of the vitamin is synthesis of cholecalciferol in the skin from cholesterol. This is accomplished through a chemical reaction that requires sun exposure, specifically ultraviolet (UV) B radiation.

For your body to produce its own vitamin D, it needs cholecalciferol, cholesterol, and UV energy from sunlight. In its original form, vitamin D isn't useful to the body. To become biologically active, it must be converted by the liver and kidneys into either calcifediol (from cholecalciferol) or 25-hydroxyergocalciferol (25[OH]D) from ergocalciferol.

Calcidediol is then further refined into calcitriol, which circulates as a hormone in the blood. It helps regulate the concentrations of calcium and phosphate, promotes the healthy growth and remodeling of bone, and helps with cell growth, neuromuscular and immune functions, and inflammation reduction.

A vitamin D-deficient diet in conjunction with inadequate sun exposure is associated with a host of problems, including fatigue, muscle spasms and twitching, cardiovascular disease, and osteomalacia (softening of the bones). It is also strongly associated with dementia and Alzheimer's. Remarkably, the vast majority of the human population has hypovitaminosis D, or vitamin D deficiency.[1]

> The biochemical actions of vitamin D and the mechanisms underlying Alzheimer's pathology overlap significantly, making this "super vitamin" exceptionally useful in the battle against dementia.

As diurnal (daytime-active) mammals, humans have evolved such that certain aspects of our biology depend on solar exposure. In a very real way and at a cellular level, our bodies rely on the sun. Sunlight syncs our circadian rhythms and, as we have discussed, triggers the chemical reaction in our skin by which vitamin D is made.

Considering how important vitamin D is to our bodies, a deficiency has damaging effects. In exploring the actions of vitamin D on overall health and specific cellular processes, scientists have discovered that it plays much bigger role than previously imagined. This "supervitamin," it turns out, affects a wide variety of processes and mechanisms throughout the body that together sustain balanced good health.

> There is increasing evidence that aging is not a singular process; rather, aging is driven by a host of cellular processes, all of which are regulated—to some extent—by vitamin D.

Increasing evidence suggests that aging is not a singular process; rather, aging is driven by a host of cellular processes such as inflammation, DNA damage or impaired transcription, oxidative stress, mitochondrial dysfunction, an inability to eliminate the metabolic byproducts of normal metabolism, decreased production of neurotrophic factors (proteins responsible for the growth, survival, and maintenance of neurons), and changes in cell-to-cell signaling. What is remarkable about all of these processes is that every single one is regulated by vitamin D.[2] What is even more remarkable is the fact that the actions of vitamin D and the mechanisms of Alzheimer's overlap significantly, making vitamin D an exceptionally useful ally in the prevention of and protection against dementia.[3]

In their 2012 article "Higher vitamin D dietary intake is associated with lower risk of Alzheimer's disease: a seven-year follow-up," Annweiler and colleagues noted that vitamin D deficiency is associated with cognitive decline in older adults.[4] They sought to determine whether the dietary intake of vitamin D was an independent predictor of the onset of dementia within seven years in women aged 75 and older. In 498 women in Toulouse, France, they found that higher vitamin D dietary intake was associated with a lower risk of Alzheimer's disease in older women.[4]

Researchers have found that baseline vitamin D concentrations in the bloodstream are strongly associated with the risk of Alzheimer's disease. As Littlejohns and others wrote in "Vitamin D and the risk of dementia and Alzheimer disease," published in 2014 in *Neurology Reviews*, people deficient in 25-hydroxyvitamin D, the major form of vitamin D in the bloodstream, may have a 51% increased risk of all-cause dementia.[5] People described as severely deficient in vitamin D may have a roughly 122% increased risk of all-cause dementia. So the more deficient in vitamin D, the greater risk for Alzheimer's disease.

The tone of recent scientific literature has changed significantly. Whereas older studies were written in cautiously optimistic terms (e.g. "vitamin D may be linked to Alzheimer's" or "may play a role in brain health"), recent studies have adopted a much more assertive stance on the topic. The connection between vitamin D and Alzheimer's is clear, and this knowledge is very useful for nutritional intervention.

> The connection between vitamin D and Alzheimer's is clear, and this knowledge is very useful for nutritional intervention.

Testing and Increasing Your Vitamin D Levels

I recommend taking a blood test to see if you have a vitamin D deficiency. A deficiency can easily be corrected. A supplementation schedule is included at the end of this chapter.

You can adjust your diet to include more sources of vitamin D, including fatty fish (tuna, mackerel, and salmon), foods fortified with vitamin D (some dairy products, orange juice, soy milk, and cereals), beef liver, cheese, and egg yolks. Vitamin D supplements are another option and are widely available.

Summary

Vitamin D is vital to your health. In humans, the most important compounds in the vitamin D group are vitamin D3 (cholecalciferol) and vitamin D2 (ergocalciferol). Much cholecalciferol is made by your body through a chemical reaction involving cholesterol and the sun's UV rays. Both types are further refined in your liver and kidneys.

As numerous studies have shown, vitamin D has an emerging relationship with Alzheimer's disease and dementia. A vitamin D deficiency, hypovitaminosis D, is associated with cognitive decline in older adults, and the greater the deficiency, the greater risk of getting Alzheimer's disease. Have your vitamin D levels checked with a simple blood test.

Key Points

- Once metabolized into its useful forms, vitamin D helps regulate calcium and phosphate, promotes bone growth, and helps with cell growth, neuromuscular and immune functions, and the reduction of inflammation.

- A vitamin D deficiency has also been linked to cognitive decline and an increased risk of Alzheimer's disease.
- If your vitamin D levels are low, adjust your and include vitamin D supplements.

Step-by-Step Action Plan to Ensure Adequate Levels of Vitamin D

Step #1: Ask your doctor to order a blood test to determine if you have a vitamin D deficiency.

Step #2: Consider taking a daily vitamin D supplement.
Recommended supplementation based on blood levels:
40–50 ng/mL: 2,000 IU
20–39 ng/mL: 5,000 IU
Less than 20 ng/mL: 10,000 IU
No need to supplement if blood levels of vitamin D are higher than 50 ng/mL.

Step #3: Consider consuming these vitamin D-rich foods:
- Fatty fish such as tuna, mackerel, and salmon
- Vitamin D-fortified dairy products, orange juice, soy milk, and cereals
- Beef liver
- Cheese
- Egg yolks

16
CURCUMIN:
ANTI-INFLAMMATORY AND ANTIOXIDANT

This book has primarily focused on the prevalence of Alzheimer's in the United States. One interesting fact is that the Indian subcontinent has the lowest prevalence of Alzheimer's disease in the world.[1] People older than 65 in some rural areas of the country have a 0.84% risk of developing the disease during their lifetime. In cities and other rural areas, the risk of Alzheimer's is 2.4%. Compare this to the rate of Alzheimer's disease in the United States— as high as a staggering 17%.

Part of the answer to these disparities can be traced to curcumin. This bright yellow powdery chemical is found primarily in turmeric, a spice and coloring agent derived from the rhizomes, or underground stems, of a plant in the ginger family. It's responsible for the yellow color of both American mustard and Indian curry. Turmeric, and therefore curcumin, is much more common in Indian cooking than in the United States, and curcumin has a long history as a traditional healing remedy in many parts of the world.

> Curcumin, a simple, inexpensive powder that has been used in traditional Indian and Chinese medicine for centuries, possesses attributes that protect against brain aging through multiple pathways.

Though this remedy has been around for generations, science has recently begun to research the folk wisdom that curcumin may prevent changes in the brain that lead to Alzheimer's. In studies of animals, it is linked to inhibition of the formation of both beta-amyloid clusters and tau tangles. Researchers have discovered that curcumin reduces oxidative damage and beta-amyloid buildup in a transgenic mouse. In vitro studies have corroborated this finding.[2]

In humans, particularly in adults susceptible to Alzheimer's disease, researchers are studying whether curcumin can improve brain function and memory. One trial found that daily curcumin doses not only prevented deterioration but also improved memory performance. Daily curcumin was compared with placebo in participants for 18 months. Based on positive cognitive outcomes, the researchers hypothesized that daily oral curcumin consumption results in less accumulation of beta-amyloid plaques, particularly in the amygdala and hypothalamus. This finding is key, because the amygdala is intricately involved in memory processing, emotions, and decision making. In addition, neurofibrillary degeneration in the hypothalamus affects neurons that block the function of cortical regions involved in Alzheimer's disease.[3]

Anti-inflammatory Properties

More than 1,300 studies have shown that curcumin has a range of health benefits, protecting against cancer cell proliferation and inflammation.

More than 1,300 studies have shown that curcumin has a range of health benefits, protecting against cancer cell proliferation and inflammation. Its anti-inflammatory effects may be key to its treatment potential for Alzheimer's disease. Inflammation causes a chain reaction that contributes to Alzheimer's. While some amyloid is commonly found in healthy brains, inflammation has a dramatic effect on the development of the toxic beta-amyloid. Inflammation may also cause tangling of the long fibers of the tau protein that serve as scaffolding. Tangling of these fibers not only kills cells but also decreases the activity of remaining cells by setting up roadblocks that interfere with cell communication. Because of inflammation, a toxic process may start years before Alzheimer's disease symptoms appear. Indeed, one of curcumin's most exciting effects is its ability to reduce, prevent, and stop inflammation.

An anti-inflammatory is a substance or treatment that reduces inflammation or swelling. A vital part of the body's natural immune response, inflammation is the body's attempt to defend itself against foreign invaders such as viruses and bacteria, heal itself after injury, and repair damaged tissue. Biochemical processes release proteins called cytokines, which summon the body's immune cells, hormones, and nutrients to repair the damage. White blood cells rush to the injured area and ingest germs, dead or damaged cells, and other foreign materials. Swelling occurs because fluid accompanies the white blood cells, hormones, and nutrients.

Thanks to its anti-inflammatory and antioxidant characteristics, curcumin protects neurons against the effects of chronic inflammation and slows the progression of Alzheimer's through the reduction of free radical damage.

Chronic inflammation can occur when the body sends repeated inflammatory response signals to a perceived internal threat that does not require an inflammatory response. In these cases, the white blood cells arrive on the scene but have nothing to do and nowhere to go. This leads to longer-lasting health issues due to the constant present of unwanted inflammation.

This is the case with Alzheimer's disease. In the brain, the "security system" cells, called microglia, remain inactive until switched on by an intruder or disease. When these cells are activated, they recognize the characteristic amyloid plaques as dangerous and attack them as they would an infection. But unlike bacteria that can be vanquished, the plaques remain as a persistent irritant. In the conflict that simmers between microglia and plaques, noxious chemicals, including peroxide and cytokines, are released. Healthy brain cells can be caught in the conflict and damaged. The result is long-term inflammation that adversely affects normal brain function. Treatment with an anti-inflammatory like curcumin can alleviate the toxic effects on brain cells caused by chronic inflammation.

Antioxidant Properties

Adrian Lopresti, a clinical psychologist who has studied the effectiveness of curcumin in randomized trials, observed, "Curcumin can influence several mechanisms in the body; in particular, it is a powerful anti-inflammatory and antioxidant."[4] As an antioxidant, it relieves oxidative stress, which causes damage to the brain linked with aging.

> As an antioxidant, curcumin relieves oxidative stress, which causes damage to the brain linked with aging.

Aging of the brain involves a battle against injuries accumulated over the decades. A major injury is oxidative stress, the inability to protect against reactive oxygen species. It is an imbalance between the creation of free radicals and the body's ability to heal or detoxify their harmful effects. Reducing free radicals in the body or decreasing their

> Reducing free radicals in the body or decreasing their rate of production may diminish cellular damage and delay aging, which is great news for prevention of dementia.

rate of production may diminish cellular damage and delay aging, which is great news for prevention of dementia. Antioxidants can suppress the formation of free radicals, scavenge to remove them before they do damage, and repair damage once it has been done.

The good news is that curcumin scavenges for free radicals. Studies have shown that curcumin decreases oxidative damage and suppresses harmful reactive changes in brain cells in response to damage to the central nervous system. In this way, curcumin reduces both oxidative damage and beta-amyloid plaque levels.[5] Thanks to these characteristics, curcumin both protects neurons against the effects of aging and slows the progression of Alzheimer's disease.

One reason that a cure for Alzheimer's disease has been elusive is that many mechanisms, not just one, appear to contribute to it. Curcumin is a potent defense against Alzheimer's disease because of its properties as both an anti-inflammatory and an antioxidant. The two processes are intricately related. In more technical terms, the stimulation of free radicals caused by oxidation then induces the production of pro-inflammatory cytokines. This interconnected loop, which can lead to neuron damage, requires both anti-inflammatory and antioxidant treatment in order to be properly addressed. A substance like curcumin, proven to have both anti-inflammatory and antioxidant abilities, shows promise for effective treatment.

How to Take Curcumin

Although curcumin has clear therapeutic value, one challenge to receiving its benefits is its bioavailability, or the proportion of curcumin that actually enters the circulation when you take it. In short, the way curcumin is ingested affects the way it is distributed and used in the body. A capsule of curcumin may be absorbed, but that does not necessarily mean it is available to the brain.

Since curcumin exists naturally in turmeric, and traditional Indian curry dishes boost the bioavailability of curcumin, eating curry dishes is an excellent way to consume curcumin in your diet. This may be the simplest—and most enjoyable—way to incorporate curcumin in your life.

Aside from eating more curry, researchers are studying how we can

Since curcumin exists naturally in turmeric, and traditional Indian curry dishes boost the bioavailability of curcumin, eating curry dishes is an excellent way to consume curcumin in your diet.

derive maximum benefits from supplementation with curcumin. One of these ways involves mixing it with other compounds. When it is combined with piperine, a major ingredient of black pepper, curcumin bioavailability increases by 2000% at 45 minutes.[6]

More than one-thousand studies have documented the health benefits of curcumin. In animal and human studies, researchers are finding that curcumin protects against the neurodegeneration that is the basis of Alzheimer's. Curcumin's anti-inflammatory and antioxidant effects are important to diminish the toxic protein buildup in Alzheimer's disease. Alzheimer's is a multifactorial disease. A simple, inexpensive powder that has been used in Indian and Chinese medicine for centuries, curcumin has attributes that protect the aging brain in many ways.

Summary

The Indian subcontinent has the lowest rate of Alzheimer's disease in the world. Part of the answer may be curcumin, an ingredient in Indian cuisine that people tend to eat much more often than in the United States. Curcumin can prevent changes in the brain that lead to the development of Alzheimer's. Daily doses of curcumin have been shown to improve cognitive performance. It appears to break down accumulations of beta-amyloid plaques in the amygdala and hippocampus. Curcumin may also help reduce damage from Alzheimer's because of its anti-inflammatory properties. In addition, by functioning as an antioxidant, curcumin helps reduce free radicals and the damage they cause through oxidative stress. Curcumin simultaneously interrupts several mechanisms that lead to Alzheimer's disease.

Key Points

- Curcumin reduces oxidative damage and beta-amyloid deposits in mice.
- Daily curcumin doses over 18 months not only prevented deterioration in memory but even improved memory performance.

- Curcumin helps alleviate toxic effects on brain cells caused by inflammatory reactions to plaques and tangles.
- The best way to take curcumin is with other compounds and foods, including black pepper.

Step-by-Step Action Plan to Consume Curcumin

Step #1: Prepare and eat curry dishes, which contain turmeric and, therefore, curcumin.

Step #2: Consider bioavailable curcumin supplements, including:

1. Meriva®, 150 mg twice a day
2. Theracurmin®, 90 mg twice a day
3. Addition of Bioperine, 5 mg, to curcumin supplements dramatically increases bioavailability. The dose is 90 mg, twice a day.

17
NAC PROTECTS ALONG
MULTIPLE PATHWAYS

Like curcumin, N-acetylcysteine (NAC) has powerful antioxidant effects. Levels of NAC diminish at an early stage of Alzheimer's disease, and diminished levels correlate with worse cognitive functioning.[1] NAC is an amino acid, or a building block of protein. It is also a precursor of glutathione, the most powerful antioxidant the body produces. Glutathione is an antioxidant and, as such, can eliminate potentially harmful free radicals in the body. It can also regulate neurotransmitter levels both inside cells and throughout brain tissues.

Aging often depletes antioxidants in the human body, leading to oxidative stress and damage to DNA, proteins, and lipids. Oxidative stress is a primary mechanism of cognitive change, leading to memory loss and, eventually, other aspects of thinking and awareness, causing confusion and mood swings. People with Alzheimer's disease have high levels of oxidative stress.

NAC scavenges free radicals and supports the body's natural defense system. It also lowers levels of pro-inflammatory cytokines. This is critical in protecting against Alzheimer's, as the hippocampus, center of memory formation and preservation in the brain, is particularly vulnerable

NAC, in combination with other nutrients, offers what is currently our best hope for preventing and treating the cognitive declines associated with Alzheimer's disease.

to inflammation. NAC also confers protection through other mechanisms. It modulates the pathways of neurotransmitters, including glutamate and dopamine. NAC enhances mitochondrial function and improves the growth and integrity of neural cells. In addition, NAC restores synaptic plasticity.[2]

Studies in mice highlight the neuroprotection properties of NAC. Mice that overproduce beta-amyloid at about six to eight months were studied to determine if antioxidant treatment with NAC could improve their cognition. The mice that consumed chow supplemented with NAC showed a greater ability to find their way through a maze in order to avoid shock and to press the correct lever to receive a food reward. The oxidative stress level in 12-month-old mice was reduced by NAC doses to levels no different from those in four-month-old mice. The researchers concluded that oxidative stress led to poor cognitive performance in the older mice and found that NAC offered therapeutic benefits.[3]

Research in humans also reveals that NAC can protect against cognitive decline. A study of 34 patients with mild cognitive impairment found that people performed better on tests of memory and other cognitive functions after taking an NAC supplement.[4] The researchers concluded that NAC lowered the participants' oxidative stress and diminished their memory impairments.[4] The scientists speculate that NAC and other nutritional modifications are most helpful when initiated before cognitive decline has grown severe and brain atrophy has begun.

> By scavenging free radicals and supporting the body's natural defense systems, the antioxidant molecule NAC protects against the cellular damage of oxidative stress in Alzheimer's disease.

In a study of people without dementia, NAC was compared with placebo.[5] Two weeks after they began the supplement, patients showed improved memory, language initiation, and executive function. Those on NAC had significantly higher scores on measures of cognitive performance at two weeks. Further improvements were observed three and six months after the study began.[5]

NAC has also been studied in patients with dementia. In a study of participants with Alzheimer's disease, those taking NAC performed better three and six months after the study began on nearly all measures of cognitive and executive function.[6] Statistically significant improvements were seen for several tasks, including letter fluency and figure reproduction.

At least four studies have assessed the value of NAC as part of a nutritional supplement, sometimes called a nutraceutical formulation. A study of more than three-hundred participants showed that participants taking this formulation performed much better than the group on placebo on tests of cognitive ability and executive function. Improvements in memory were visible three and six months after dosage began. Because of the improved cognitive abilities of participants taking NAC, the researchers felt it would be unethical to continue randomly assigning a study group to placebo; all participants were therefore given the nutraceutical formulation. A study on NAC administration as part of a multi-compound formulation found the subjects performed better on general cognition, executive function, processing speed, and visuospatial reasoning than the placebo group.[7] Researchers conducting these studies have observed that, in addition to improving cognitive performance, NAC is well tolerated. The investigators emphasize the importance of beginning the nutritional supplementation at the onset of, or even before, cognitive decline begins in order to attain maximum effectiveness.

Effects on mild cognitive impairment and Alzheimer's disease appear to be more robust when NAC is part of a combined treatment. This, however, makes it challenging to isolate exactly which benefits are conferred by the NAC itself. More studies will undoubtedly shed light on NAC's specific benefits. In the meantime, it is clearly an important addition to a nutraceutical prevention and treatment for mild cognitive decline and Alzheimer's. A recent expert review concluded that antioxidants such as NAC should be given along with B Vitamins as part of treatment for patients with dementia.[8]

One challenge with NAC is that it has low bioavailability, which means that ingesting the supplement does not ensure that its benefits reach the brain. It must be able to cross the blood-brain barrier. Bioavailability of

NAC improves when it is taken as a derivative like N-acetylcysteine amide, which has a higher permeability through cell and mitochondrial membranes.[1]

> Bioavailability of NAC improves when it is taken as a derivative like N-acetylcysteine amide, which has a higher permeability through cell and mitochondrial membranes.

Part of the reason drug treatments for Alzheimer's don't work is that the disease involves interrelated abnormalities. Also, Alzheimer's develops slowly, and by the time the first symptoms appear, it may be too late to change its course. The pharmaceutical companies' formulations, which target just one mechanism, have been entirely ineffective at changing the devastating course of the disease.

Nutritional supplementation promotes brain health and targets the damage through multiple pathways. NAC regulates dopamine and glutamate, balances enzymes and signaling systems, enhances mitochondrial function, controls inflammatory response, and promotes neural growth and integrity. Considerable evidence exists that increased oxidative stress, inflammation, mitochondrial dysfunction, and cell death are linked to cognitive deterioration.

Therapeutic Mechanisms of NAC

> NAC offers the best hope for preventing and treating the cognitive decline associated with Alzheimer's disease.

- Antioxidant production
- Neurotransmitter modulation
- Inflammatory regulation
- Mitochondrial energy
- Neurotrophic support

In combination with other nutrients, NAC can reduce the severity of cognitive changes. It offers the best hope for preventing and treating the cognitive decline associated with Alzheimer's disease.

Summary

NAC confers both antioxidant and anti-inflammatory protection as well as modulation of pathways of the important neurotransmitters glutamate and dopamine. It enhances mitochondrial function, improves growth of neural cells, and restores synaptic plasticity. Studies in mice and people with and without dementia demonstrate NAC's beneficial effects on cognitive decline.

Key Points

- Several studies demonstrate the positive cognitive effects of NAC as a nutritional supplement.
- The effects appear to be more robust when NAC is part of a combined treatment.
- Because of low bioavailability, NAC should be taken as a derivative like N-acetylcysteine amide.
- NAC affects the development of Alzheimer's disease through several therapeutic pathways, including anti-inflammatory and antioxidant reduction, neurotransmitter modulation, and neurotrophic and mitochondrial support.

Step-by-Step Action Plan to Consume Adequate NAC

Step #1: Take the dietary supplement N-acetylcysteine (NAC) 600 mg–2,000 mg a day.

Step #2: Consider a combination supplement with lithium, NAC, and B vitamins.
- Luma (JayMac Pharmaceuticals) – A multinutrient Alzheimer's prevention supplement with 2.5 mg of lithium orotate per tablet (lumaforlife.com)

18
BRAIN FOODS:
BLUEBERRIES, GRAPE SEED, AND GREEN TEA

Blueberries

Certain foods offer some protection against cognitive decline. Blueberries, which grow in temperate climates all over the world, provide excellent nutrition and enhance health. These benefits come from both the larger highbush form and the smaller lowbush, or wild, blueberry. Scientists have long known that blueberries have health benefits, as they appear to confer protection against heart disease and cancer.

Blueberries have a high flavonoid content which, in addition to causing the vivid colors in many fruits and vegetables, help maintain healthy metabolism. They are powerful antioxidants, which we've learned is an important preventive nutritional tool against Alzheimer's disease. Their capacity as antioxidants comes mainly from their high content of antho-cyanins, a type of flavonoid. These are water-soluble pigments that may be red, purple, or blue. (The "cyan" in "anthocyanins" comes from the Greek *kuaneos*, for dark blue.)

As antioxidants, blueberries prevent or neutralize the damaging effects of free radicals. In addition to antioxidant properties, flavonoids also work as anti-inflammatories. As we know, these two characteristics work together in important ways to undo oxidation and inflammation in the brain. Researchers have found that blueberries provide

> Certain dietary flavonoids—like those present in blueberries, grape seeds, and green tea—appear to have neuroprotective effects.

significant benefits in improving symptoms of metabolic syndrome and other cardiovascular risk factors related to obesity, including high blood pressure. Both animal and human studies have demonstrated these effects. Blueberries also help improve brain health. The anthocyanins in blueberries have been associated with increased neuronal signaling in brain centers, mediating memory function, improving disposal of glucose, and enhancing hippocampal plasticity. These benefits protect against neurodegeneration, another key to dementia prevention.

In addition to their anti-inflammatory and antioxidant capabilities, blueberries have also been shown improve memory in older adults. A 2010 study conducted by Krikorian and colleagues demonstrated the benefits of wild blueberry juice among adults with early memory changes. The study subjects who drank blueberry juice rather than a placebo beverage exhibited significantly better memory performance than those drinking placebo. This was the first human trial exploring the potential benefit of blueberry supplementation on neurocognitive function in older adults at increased risk for dementia.[1]

A later trial conducted by the same researchers assessed the effects of consuming blueberries by using both memory tests and MRIs.[2] The participants who received freeze-dried blueberry powder once a day for 16 weeks not only had improved memory and better word retrieval than before the study began, their MRIs registered increased brain activity. These positive changes were not present in the group that received placebo powder.[1]

A recent study demonstrated that participants aged 60 to 75 who were given blueberries instead of a blueberry placebo performed better than controls on several tests of cognitive function.[3] At baseline, at the midpoint of 45 days, and at 90 days, the subjects completed a series of balance, gait, and cognitive tests. Participants eating blueberries made fewer repetition errors on the California Verbal Learning test and achieved better results on a task-switching tests than controls.[3]

Blueberries have even been shown to reverse age-related cognitive deficits in memory in both animals and humans. Working with children aged seven to 10, researchers determined that blueberry consumption can almost immediately improve cognitive performance.[4] Children in the study were given either freeze-dried blueberry powder or placebo. Those consuming blueberry powder performed various mental tests faster and more accurately than the placebo group. The researchers concluded that blueberries can enhance executive function during challenging tasks.

Blueberries have also been shown to improve physical mobility in older people. In a study to determine whether six weeks of frozen blueberry consumption would improve functional mobility in older adults, researchers documented improvements in the blueberry group's casual walking speed and gait but not in the placebo group.[5] The researchers hypothesized that the polyphenolic compounds in blueberries lower oxidative stress and inflammation.

Supplementing your diet with blueberries can help with mobility challenges due to aging, memory, and cognition. The blueberry's properties as both an anti-inflammatory and an antioxidant explain its efficacy in preventing cognitive decline and Alzheimer's disease and even in reversing some of the disease's damaging effects. It can also counteract age-related decline in functional mobility.

> "Brain foods" are, very simply, substances from nature that have been used for millennia as medicines to boost vitality and restore health.

Grape Seed

Other foods also contain powerful flavonoids that can boost brain health and delay the onset of effects of dementia. Another food rich in flavonoids is grape seed, used since the time of the ancient Greeks to enhance health.

Grape seed extract is produced by grinding the seeds at the center of grapes and using a steam distillation process or a cold-pressing method to extract their pure compounds. Today, grape seed extract is used as a dietary supplement to reduce inflammation.

Recently, grape seed has also been shown to be a powerful weapon against oxidative stress. Moreover, the flavonoids in grape seed may have other positive effects on the aging brain. In tests in mice, grape seed extract significantly inhibited the formation of beta-amyloid protein, the plaque-forming precursor to Alzheimer's disease. For five months, a group of mice received water containing grape seed extract or water alone as a placebo treatment.[6]

> In tests in mice, grape seed extract significantly inhibited the formation of beta-amyloid protein, the plaque-forming precursor to Alzheimer's disease.

The researchers found that, compared with the mice given only water, those treated with grape seed extract had significantly less Alzheimer's disease-type cognitive deterioration. Fewer beta-amyloid plaques had formed in their brains. This evidence has been corroborated by subsequent studies in mice at an age when they would normally develop signs of Alzheimer's disease. Compared with mice given the placebo, the mice fed grape seed extract had fewer plaque clusters and demonstrated less cognitive decline. Before the onset of symptoms, the grape seed extract may have prevented or postponed plaque formation and thereby slowed cognitive deterioration associated with Alzheimer's disease.

Green Tea

Therapeutic flavonoids are also present in other foods, particularly in green tea. In a small research study, scientists demonstrated that green tea extract promoted increased brain activity.[7] The MRIs of volunteers assigned to drink a beverage containing green tea extract showed more brain activity in the prefrontal cortex, a key brain area responsible for memory processing, than the MRIs of those who drank a placebo extract.

A very large study of older Chinese subjects demonstrated the neurocognitive benefits of tea consumption.[8] In nearly one-thousand people who were cognitively intact at the beginning of the study in 2003, researchers found a significantly higher percentage of cognitive degeneration years later among those who did not drink tea. Those who drank tea had a lower risk of Alzheimer's disease.

Studies in mice have found that green tea directly affects beta-amyloid plaques. When green tea extract was added to mouse chow, beta-amyloid deposits in the brain were small and formless rather than clustered in harmful plaques.[9] The prevention of these plaques is key to delaying the damaging effects of dementia.

> When green tea extract was added to mouse chow, beta-amyloid deposits in the brain were small and formless rather than clustered in harmful plaques.

The neuroprotective effects of certain dietary flavonoids appear to include the potential to protect neurons against injury induced by neurotoxins, suppress neuroinflammation, and increase memory, learning, and cognitive function. These flavonoids inhibit cell death and promote the survival of neurons and synaptic plasticity.

Like lithium, these brain foods are nothing new. They are not complex formulations made by pharmaceutical companies but rather simple substances found in nature that have been around for a very long time.

Supplements Work Best in Combinations

Some studies are finding that using supplements in combination is preferable to using a supplement alone, and research trials adopting a combination approach show promise in both early- and late-stage Alzheimer's.[10] Though B vitamins can improve cognitive function and lower homocysteine levels, lowering homocysteine addresses only one of several pro-inflammatory mechanisms that lead to oxidative stress. Given the interdependent relationship between oxidative stress and homocysteine, it is wise to give other antioxidant supplements with B vitamins.

Summary

Eating blueberries has long been linked to health benefits. The anthocyanins in blueberries are strong antioxidants and anti-inflammatories. In addition, they lead to increased neuron signaling and enhanced hippocampal plasticity and protect against degeneration. Blueberries improve memory performance in older adults, as evidenced on both cognitive measures and MRI scans. They have been shown to reverse cognitive decline in older adults.

The flavonoid content of grape seed bolsters brain health and delays the onset of dementia. High in flavonoids, grape seed leads to increases in brain-derived neurotrophic factor (BDNF).

Flavonoids in green tea may lead to increased activity in the prefrontal cortex, a part of the brain critical for memory. Polyphenols appear to have a range of positive effects on the brain, promoting synaptic plasticity, inhibiting brain atrophy, and suppressing inflammation. The lower risk of dementia in countries where green tea is a staple suggests that Western countries would do well to increase their own consumption of green tea to protect brain health.

Key Points

- Anthocyanin gives blueberries antioxidants and anti-inflammatory abilities.
- MRIs of patients in a study showed that those who ate blueberries had increased brain activity, unlike those on placebo.
- Grape seed extract has been shown to improve cognitive function in mice.

- In a very large study of older Chinese people without cognitive symptoms, those who drank green tea had a lower risk of cognitive decline than those who did not regularly drink green tea.

Step-by-Step Action Plan to Incorporate More Brain Foods into Your Diet

Step #1: Consider consuming more blueberries, grapes, and green tea in your diet.

Step #2: Take the dietary supplement CurcumaSorb Mind, 2 capsules a day (Pure Encapsulations). This supplement combines bioavailable curcumin with a blend of blueberry and grape seed extract (pureencapsulations.com).

PART 5
FOOD FOR THOUGHT

19
A GOLDEN PUBLIC HEALTH INTERVENTION

James Phelps, editor of *Psychiatric Times*, posed the question as the title of a 2016 article: "Lithium for Alzheimer Prevention: What Are We Waiting For?"[1] He envisioned these scenarios:

Imagine if:

- Animal studies conducted by a big drug company showed that a substance delivering significant benefits in preventing neurodegeneration, reducing two major symptoms that accompany Alzheimer's disease: tau protein phosphorylation (tangles) and beta-amyloid plaque formation.

> "Why is there so little clamor from patients at high risk for Alzheimer's disease and their families for lithium?"
> ~Dr. James Phelps

- In a preliminary trial, their new drug inhibited these two changes in humans.
- In more than 90% of patients tested, there were no known risks or side effects.
- The drug was effective even in patients who already had early signs of Alzheimer's disease.

What would happen? A stampede! The large drug company would be flooded with demands for the humanitarian release of their new product based on the large number of adults at very high risk for Alzheimer's disease in the next decade. The demand would be high even before formal clinical trials got underway.

All these scenarios are true for lithium. Dr. Phelps concluded, "Why is there so little clamor from patients at high risk for Alzheimer's disease and their families for lithium?"[1] The relative lack of attention to lithium for Alzheimer's disease is particularly striking because such a tiny dose seems to confer benefits. And at microdoses, side effects are not an issue.

The enormous potential of lithium as a public health intervention is already crystal clear, as evidenced by the Texas Drinking Water Study referenced previously.[2] In fact, the authors of that study suggested lithiation of drinking water as a public health intervention to reduce crime, suicide, and drug dependency at the community level. The results of that study have been replicated around the world. More than 20 years later, a Japanese study researched 18 municipalities with more than a million inhabitants over five years.[3] Suicide rates were inversely correlated with lithium content in the local water supply.

In addition to these studies on drinking water levels, there is much to say about the possibilities of suicide prevention and lithium treatment, which may contribute to the rationale of drinking water lithiation. Since the 1970s, numerous international studies of lithium have documented lithium's anti-suicidal effects.[4,5] As Lewitzka and others wrote in "The suicide prevention effect of lithium: more than 20 years of evidence— a narrative review" in 2015, an early description of lithium's anti-suicidal properties was made in 1972 when Barraclough analyzed the clinical history of one-hundred people who died by suicide.[6] He concluded that as many as a fifth of these suicides may have been prevented if lithium had been used. A 2017 study of 50,000 patients with bipolar disorder showed similar promise and concluded that up to 10 percent of attempted or completed suicides could have been avoided for bipolar patients if they had been treated with lithium.[7] Lithium's health benefits include suicide prevention, which must also be considered when we imagine its possibilities as a public health intervention.

> The prospect of a golden public health intervention is before us. What *are* we waiting for?

Dr. Lars Vedel Kessing et al. explored the connection between lithium in drinking water and the incidence of dementia.[8] Reporting in *JAMA Psychiatry* in 2017, he revealed that, in a study of more than 800,000 individuals, those with dementia had been exposed to less lithium than controls. This nationwide Danish study calculated lithium content in water samples, tracked the addresses of each participant, and calculated exposures since 1986.

In an editorial that accompanied the release of the study results, Drs. John McGrath and Michael Berk wrote, "The prospect that a relatively safe, simple, and cheap intervention (i.e. optimizing lithium concentrations in the drinking water) could lead to the primary prevention of dementia is a tantalizing prospect. . . In the spirit of alchemy, could we convert lithium, a simple metal used as a mood stabilizer, into a golden public health intervention that could prevent dementia?"[9] They concluded that even a marginal reduction in the dementia incidence would yield major societal and economic gains.

> "In the spirit of alchemy, could we convert lithium, a simple metal used as a mood stabilizer, into a golden public health intervention that could prevent dementia?"
> ~Drs. John McGrath and Michael Berk

Dr. Anna Fels, the psychiatrist who labelled lithium a Cinderella drug, speculated, "Should we all take a bit of lithium?"[10] She continued, "What if microdose lithium were again part of our standard nutritional fare? What if it were added back to soft drinks or popular vitamin brands or even put into the water supply? The research to date strongly suggests that suicide levels would be reduced, and even perhaps other violent acts. And maybe the dementia rate would decline."

Lithium affects many biological pathways linked to progressive neurodegenerative disorders. It exerts effects on mechanisms that involve intracellular calcium glutamate excitotoxicity, apoptosis, inflammation, and oxidative stress. It increases synaptic plasticity and inhibits GSK3, which plays a role in the formation of tau tangles. In addition to preventing the neuron degeneration of dementia, it confers other neuropsychiatric benefits. It is linked to reductions in suicide, homicide, and other violent crime. A low level of lithium in the water supply is relatively safe, simple, and inexpensive to implement. The prospect of a golden public health intervention is before us. What *are* we waiting for?

Summary

The relative lack of attention to lithium is especially striking, as such a tiny dose confers benefits. The efficacy in small doses reduces concern about safety and side effects. Counties in Texas where the drinking water had naturally occurring lithium had lower rates of suicide, murder, and drug abuse than other counties where the water supply contained no lithium. These findings have been replicated in other areas around the world. In 2017, a Danish study reported that rates of dementia were higher in areas where drinking water contained no lithium than in areas with lithium in the water supply. The researchers suggest that lithium has potential as a "golden public health intervention." A low level of lithium in drinking water would be safe, simple, and easy to implement.

Key Points

- Data published in 2017 from 800,000 individuals in Denmark indicated that those with Alzheimer's disease had been exposed to less lithium in the water supply than those without the disease.
- Lithium shows immense promise as a suicide prevention measure for certain mood disorders.
- Lithiation of the water supply is a feasible public health intervention that could yield astounding social and economic benefits.

20
CONCLUSION:
LITHIUM AND HAPPIER AGING

We began this book by discussing the failure of the pharmaceutical industry to find a way to prevent or cure Alzheimer's disease despite billions of dollars of investment. As different theories to explain the brain damage caused by Alzheimer's have been proposed through the years, medications have been developed based on each theory in order to target a particular hypothesized pathway of the disease. Clinical trials sponsored by pharmaceutical companies throughout the world have enrolled thousands of patients, yet none of the drugs have met criteria for effectiveness.

That we have no pharmaceutical cure for Alzheimer's disease is certainly not because of lack of effort. Rather, Alzheimer's has proven to be elusive to treat because of its complexity and the intricate interrelation of brain processes that scientists still do not fully understand. The most common explanation is that Alzheimer's results from both the accumulation of beta-amyloid plaques and that neurofibrillary tangles from hyperphosphorylated tau proteins kill brain cells. Inflammatory changes from the body's attempt to clear beta-amyloid plaques may be a contributing cause. With so many factors implicated in

> Alzheimer's has proven to be elusive to treat because of its complexity and the intricate interrelation of brain processes that scientists still do not fully understand.

the disease, a drug targeting only one of these damaging processes could leave the others continue unchecked.

Pharmaceutical trials from drug companies around the world seem to reveal a pattern of hopeful early promise followed by major expenditures of time and money and, finally, disappointing results. Drug research continues, driven by desire to alleviate this devastating disease that is growing in prevalence. Also, of course, the financial reward for finding a pharmaceutical cure will be enormous. We are likely to continue to hear reports of the latest new prospect to cure Alzheimer's disease, but we will have to wait till any drug has overcome the hurdles that have defeated all previous candidates.

Instead of waiting, the best treatment for Alzheimer's disease is prevention. The best way to protect against the damage caused by this disease is to promote the health of the brain. Instead of focusing on 1 possible disease pathway and trying to arrest it, we can use low-dose lithium and additional supplements that foster the health of brain cells and forestall the damaging mechanisms that may be involved in the cell atrophy that is Alzheimer's disease. The studies cited in these chapters have shown that lithium and other neuroprotective supplements can prevent or stop the formation of beta-amyloid plaques, prevent inflammation, balance neurotransmitters, and exert antioxidant effects to minimize the damage caused by free radicals. The most important of these supplements is lithium. Others, including vitamins B6, B12, folate, curcumin, and certain foods, contribute to protecting the brain as well. These supplements—at recommended doses and over a long enough time—can improve the health of the brain. This, in turn, enhances quality of life and even reduces damage from Alzheimer's disease.

Lithium offers a promising and inexpensive route of prevention thanks to the research into how it helps protect against neurodegeneration. It is thoroughly studied, proven effective in addressing the many factors that lead to dementia, and easily accessible. We know that the economic, personal, and social consequences of Alzheimer's disease are devastating, and I truly believe that incorporating low-dose lithium as well as other nutritional and lifestyle changes is the most effective and affordable preventive option available.

And though we have focused on introducing lithium as a key preventive supplement, it is important to remember that how we live is as impactful as the supplements we take. Emerging research shows that lifestyle factors in themselves protect brain health and may postpone death. We have long known, for instance, that social connections improve psychological health. But new research reveals that active involvement with other people protects physical health as well. We know this from lived experience, too, that when we are well connected to our peers and loved ones, we are more likely to experience joy, purpose, and health.

> When we are well connected to our peers and loved ones, we are more likely to experience joy, purpose, and health.

One of the most promising avenues to discover the influence of lifestyle on health is to follow in the steps of Dan Buettner, who, for more than two decades, has studied areas on the planet where people live the longest and healthiest lives.[1] Citing evidence from Danish twin studies that genetics contribute about 25% to longevity, he focuses on the 75% contributed by lifestyle. Instead of looking at the lives of individuals, who might have a genetic predisposition to long life, he explores longevity pockets to find the impact of lifestyle. The first pocket he found was the island of Okinawa, where the rate of centenarians is three times the rate in the United States. Moreover, Okinawans have one-fifth the rate of heart disease and live, on average, seven years longer than Americans. In addition to Okinawa, Buettner has found such pockets in the Barbagia region of Sardinia in Italy, Loma Linda in California, and the Nicoya peninsula in Costa Rica. Here is a distillation of the wisdom for healthy aging that Buettner found by studying these groups[1]:

- Move naturally. Exercise, but as part of your daily routine, not necessarily by working out on a treadmill.
- Know and discover your purpose. Use this as motivation to live a life of meaning and dignity.
- Shed stress wherever possible.
- Eat a little less. Stop eating when you are 80% full.
- Eat less meat.
- Drink in moderation or not at all.
- Have faith. Collective organizing around a shared belief system is more important than support of a particular religious institution.
- Put families first.
- Stay social. Make sure your social network supports healthy behaviors.

Indeed, our own perceptions of aging serve as a lens through which we interpret changes and attribute their causes. Dread of aging and resentment of changes it brings releases a cascade of negative energy that can make the dreaded outcomes more real and significant. Do your best to reflect on and embrace the natural effects of aging. Aging is inevitable, and the suffering we so often associate with it is avoidable. We are all fortunate to live in exciting times when new research from the field of neuroscience is expanding our knowledge of physical and mental health. We also have greater access to ways to maintain and improve our health, particularly the health of our brains.

> We are all fortunate to live in exciting times when new research from the field of neuroscience is expanding our knowledge of physical and mental health.

As yet, we have no cure for conditions like Alzheimer's disease. But, by focusing on protecting and enriching the health of our brains, we can postpone its appearance, prevent unwanted suffering, and even reverse some of its effects. Meanwhile, we can strive to master the balance of a healthy connection to our family, friends, and environment.

I wish you a long and healthy life!

Step-by-Step Action Plan for a Long and Healthy Life[1]

Step #1: Move naturally. Exercise, but as part of your daily routine.

Step #2: Know and discover a purpose. Use this as motivation to live a life with meaning.

Step #3: Shed stress wherever possible.

Step #4: Eat a little less. Stop eating when you are 80% full.

Step #5: Eat less meat.

Step #6: Drink in moderation or not at all.

Step #7: Have faith. Collective organizing around a shared belief system is more important than support of a particular religious institution.

Step #8: Put families first.

Step #9: Stay social. Make sure your social network supports healthy behaviors.

Integrative Medicine for Alzheimer's
Action Plan Summary

Low-Dose Lithium

Step #1: To determine if you are deficient in lithium, order a hair tissue mineral analysis kit from Great Plains Laboratory (greatplainslaboratory.com) or a urine test from ZRT Laboratory (zrtlab.com).*

Step #2: Start lithium supplementation:
- Lithium orotate, 2.5 mg a day, or liquid lithium citrate, 1.0 mg a day
- Luma (JayMac Pharmaceuticals) – A multinutrient Alzheimer's prevention supplement with 2.5 mg of lithium orotate per tablet (lumaforlife.com)
- Liquid lithium (Pure Encapsulations) – A liquid preparation of lithium citrate, 2 mg (pureencapsulations.com).

*Lithium deficiency is not recognized by the Food and Nutrition Board of the Institute of Medicine in the National Academy of Sciences.

Lowering Homocysteine

Step #1: Ask your doctor to order blood tests for vitamin B12, folate, and a genetic test, usually a cheek swab for the MTHFR gene.

Step #2: If your doctor tells you that you have elevated homocysteine levels (over 11 μmol/L) then you must determine if the low level is related to B12 deficiency or folate deficiency.

Step #3: If deficient in vitamin B12 (blood test values are under 500 ng/mL) take at least 5,000 mcg of methylcobalamin daily. If your level is under 400 ng/mL talk with your doctor about vitamin B12 injections.

Step #4: If you have any of the genetic variants on the MTHFR gene take L-methylfolate 1-5 mg/day.

Step #5: There are nutritional supplements that combine all the nutrients that lower homocysteine, folate, vitamin B6 and vitamin B12.
- Luma (JayMac Pharmaceuticals) – A multinutrient Alzheimer's prevention supplement with 2.5 mg of lithium orotate per tablet (lumaforlife.com)

Vitamin D

Step #1: Ask your doctor to order a blood test to determine if you have a vitamin D deficiency.

Step #2: Consider taking a daily vitamin D supplement.
  Recommended supplementation based on blood levels:
  40–50 ng/mL: 2,000 IU
  20–39 ng/mL: 5,000 IU
  Less than 20 ng/mL: 10,000 IU
No need to supplement if blood levels of vitamin D are higher than 50 ng/mL.

Step #3: Consider consuming these vitamin D-rich foods:
- Fatty fish such as tuna, mackerel, and salmon
- Vitamin D-fortified dairy products, orange juice, soy milk, and cereals
- Beef liver
- Cheese
- Egg yolks

Curcumin

Step #1: Prepare and eat curry dishes, which contain turmeric and, therefore, curcumin.

Step #2: Consider bioavailable curcumin supplements, including:
- Meriva®, 150 mg twice a day
- Theracurmin®, 90 mg twice a day
- Addition of Bioperine, 5 mg, to curcumin supplements dramatically increases bioavailability. The dose is 90 mg twice a day.

NAC

Step #1: Take the dietary supplement N-acetylcysteine (NAC) 600 mg–2,000 mg a day.

Brain Foods

Step #1: Consider consuming more blueberries, grapes, and green tea in your diet.

Step #2: Take the dietary supplement CurcumaSorb Mind, two capsules a day (Pure Encapsulations). This supplement combines bioavailable curcumin with a blend of blueberry and grape seed extract (pureencapsulations.com).

A Meaningful Life[1]

Step #1: Move naturally. Exercise, but as part of your daily routine.

Step #2: Know and discover a purpose. Use this as motivation to live a life with meaning.

Step #3: Shed stress wherever possible.

Step #4: Eat a little less. Stop eating when you are 80% full.

Step #5: Eat less meat.

Step #6: Drink in moderation or not at all.

Step #7: Have faith. Collective organizing around a shared belief system is more important than support of a particular religious institution.

Step #8: Put families first.

Step #9: Stay social. Make sure your social network supports healthy behaviors.

DISCLAIMER

The information presented in this book has not been evaluated or approved by the U.S. Food and Drug Administration. The products discussed in this book are not intended to diagnose, treat, cure, or prevent any disease.

The information reviewed in this book is designed to provide information on currently available research on low-dose lithium. This book is not intended, nor should it be used, as a substitute for the medical advice of physicians. The reader should regularly consult a physician in matters relating to his/her health and particularly with respect to any symptoms that may require diagnosis or medical attention. Nutritional supplements should be taken under the supervision of a health care professional.

Warning: Lithium should not be taken by pregnant or lactating women. Low-dose lithium is not a replacement for prescription lithium for patients with bipolar disorder. Do not take lithium if you have thyroid or kidney disease. Do not exceed 5.0 mg a day of lithium without being monitored by a health professional.

ABOUT THE AUTHOR

A pioneer in the field of integrative medicine, James M. Greenblatt, MD, has treated patients since 1988. After receiving his medical degree and completing his psychiatry residency at George Washington University, Dr. Greenblatt completed a fellowship in child and adolescent psychiatry at Johns Hopkins Medical School. Dr. Greenblatt currently serves as the Chief Medical Officer at Walden Behavioral Care in Waltham, MA and serves as an Assistant Clinical Professor of Psychiatry at Tufts University School of Medicine and Dartmouth College Geisel School of Medicine.

An acknowledged integrative medicine expert, educator, and author, Dr. Greenblatt has lectured internationally on the scientific evidence for nutritional interventions in psychiatry and mental illness. Through three decades of practice and research, Dr. Greenblatt has been a leading contributor to the revolution of patients and families seeking individualized care and offers evidence-based approaches toward nuanced and integrative recovery.

In April of 2017, Dr. Greenblatt was inducted into the Orthomolecular Medicine Hall of Fame by the International Society of Orthomolecular Medicine, which has recognized significant contributors to science and medicine who operate from the perspective of biochemical individuality and nutrition-based therapies since 2004. Dr. Greenblatt shares this honor with recognized founders in the field of integrative medicine, beginning with the pioneers of nutritional psychiatry Abram Hoffer, Linus Pauling, and Roger Williams.

His book series, *Psychiatry Redefined,* draws on his many years of experience and expertise in integrative medicine for psychiatry. Dr. Greenblatt's knowledge in the areas of biology, genetics, psychology, and nutrition as they interact in the treatment of mental illness has made him a highly sought-after speaker at national and international conferences and workshops. He currently offers online courses for professionals as well as specialized fellowship programs in the functional medicine approaches to integrative psychiatry. For more information, please visit www.JamesGreenblattMD.com.

REFERENCES

Chapter 1   The Burden of Alzheimer's

1. World Health Organization. *Dementia: A Public Health Priority.* http://apps.who.int/iris/bitstream/handle/10665/75263/97892415 64458_eng.pdf;jsessionid=4239C671DE61ABAEA2BEF44C667 C131D?sequence=1. 2012. Accessed August 12, 2018.

2. Hebert LE, Weuve J, Scherr PA, Evans DA. Alzheimer disease in the United States (2010-2050) estimated using the 2010 Census. *Neurology.* 2013;80(19):1778–1783.

3. Steenland K, Goldstein FC, Levey A, Wharton W. A meta-analysis of Alzheimer's disease comparing African-American and caucasians. *J Alzheimers Dis.* 2015;50(1):71–76.

4. Centers for Disease Control and Prevention. Health, United States, 2016. https://www.cdc.gov/nchs/data/hus/hus16.pdf#019. 2016. Accessed August 12, 2018.

5. Alzheimer's Association. *Early-Onset Dementia: A National Challenge, a Future Crisis.* Washington, D.C.: Alzheimer's Association; 2006.

6. Nuland SB. *How We Die: Reflections on Life's Final Chapter.* New York: Vintage Books; 2010.

7. Alzheimer's Association. 2018 Alzheimer's disease facts and figures. *Alzheimers Dement.* 2018;14(3):367–429.

8. Pritchard C, Mayers A, Baldwin D. Changing patterns of neurological mortality in the 10 major developed countries – 1979–2010. *Public Health.* 2013;127(4):357–368. doi: 10.1016/j.puhe.2012.12.018.

9. Alzheimer's Association. *Generation Alzheimer's: The Defining Disease of the Baby Boomers.* http://act.alz.org/site/DocServer/ ALZ_BoomersReport.pdf?docID=521. 2011. Accessed August 12, 2018.

Chapter 2   Alzheimer's and Dementia: The Progressive Stages
1. Mayo Clinic. Alzheimer's stages: How the disease progresses. Mayo Clinic. www.mayoclinic.org/diseases-conditions/alzheimers-disease/in-depth/alzheimers-stages/art-20048448. 2018. Accessed August 12, 2018.
2. Combs LM. *A Long Good-Bye and Beyond: Coping with Alzheimer's.* Wilsonville, OR: BooksPartners; 1999.

Chapter 3   Causes of Alzheimer's Disease and Death
1. Jansen WJ, Ossenkoppele R, Knol DL, et al. Prevalence of cerebral amyloid pathology in persons without dementia: a meta-analysis. *JAMA.* 2015;313(19):1924–1938. doi: 10.1001/jama.2015.4668.
2. Langbaum JB, Fleisher AS, Chen K, et al. Ushering in the study and treatment of preclinical Alzheimer disease [published online ahead of print June 11 2013]. *Nat Rev Neurol.* 2013;9(7):371–381. doi: 10.1038/nrneurol.2013.107.

Chapter 4   Dead Ends: The Search for a Drug Cure
1. Kelly BL, Ferreira A. Beta-amyloid-induced dynamin 1 degradation is mediated by N-methyl-D-aspartate receptors in hippocampal neurons. *J Biol Chem.* 2006;281(38):28079–28089.
2. Devlin H. Scientists find first drug that appears to slow Alzheimer's disease. *The Guardian.* www.theguardian.com/science/2015/jul/22/scientists-find-first-drug-slow-alzheimers-disease.
3. Cummings JL, Morstorf T, Zhong K. Alzheimer's disease drug-development pipeline: Few candidates, frequent failures. *Alzheimers Res Ther.* 2014;6(4):37.
4. Loftus P. Merck stops clinical trial of Alzheimer's drug. *Wall Street Journal.* https://www.wsj.com/articles/

merck-stops-clinical-trial-of-alzheimers-drug-1487115418. 2017. Accessed August 12, 2018.

5. Korczyn A. Why have we failed to cure Alzheimer's disease? *J Alzheimers Dis.* 2012; 29(2): 275–282. doi: 10.3233/JAD-2011-110359.

Chapter 5   An Accidental Discovery: Lithium, from Bipolar Disorder to Alzheimer's Disease

1. Schou M, Juel-Nielsen N, Strömgren E, Voldby H, Stromgren, E. The treatment of manic psychoses by the administration of lithium salts. *J Neurol Neurosurg Psychiatry.* 1954;17(4):250–60.

2. Manji HK, Moore GJ, Chen G. Lithium up regulates the cytoprotective protein Bcl-2 in the CNS in vivo: a role for neurotrophic and neuroprotective effects in manic depressive illness. *J Clin Psychiatry.* 2000;61(Suppl 9):82–96.

3. Moore GJ, Bebchuk JM, Wilds IB, Chen G, Manji HK. Lithium-induced increase in human brain grey matter. *Lancet.* 2000;356:1241–1242.

4. Gerhard T, Devanand DP, Huang C, Crystal S, Olfson M. Lithium treatment and risk for dementia in adults with bipolar disorder: Population-based cohort study. *Br J Psychiatry.* 2015;207(1):46–51.

5. Nunes PV, Forlenza, OV, Gattaz WF. Lithium and risk for Alzheimer's disease in elderly patients with bipolar disorder. *Br J Psychiatry.* 2007;190:359–360.

6. Kessing LV, Sondergard L, Forman JL, Andersen PK. Lithium treatment and risk of dementia. *Arch Gen Psychiatry.* 2008;65(11):1331–1335. doi: 10.1001/archpsyc.65.11.1331.

7. Bersani G, Quartini A, Zullo D, Iannitelli A. Potential neuroprotective effect of lithium in bipolar patients evaluated by neuropsychological assessment: preliminary results [published online ahead of print November 13 2015]. *Hum Psychopharmacol.* 2016;31(1):19–28. doi: 10.1002/hup.2510.

8. Nunes MA, Viel TA, Buck HS. Microdose lithium treatment stabilized cognitive impairment in patients with Alzheimer's disease. *Curr Alzheimer Res.* 2013;10(1):104–107.

9. Kessing LV, Gerds TA, Knudsen NN, et al. Association of lithium in drinking water with the incidence of dementia. *JAMA Psychiatry.* 2017;74(10):1005–1010. doi:10.1001/jamapsychiatry.2017.2362.

10. Fajardo VA, LeBlanc PJ, MacPherson RK. Examining the relationship between trace lithium in drinking water and the rising rates of age-adjusted Alzheimer's disease mortality in Texas. *J. Alzheimers Dis.* 2018;61(1):425–434. doi: 10.3233/JAD-170744.

11. Matsunaga S, Kishi T, Annas P, et al. Lithium as a treatment for Alzheimer's disease: A systematic review and meta-analysis. *J Alzheimers Dis.* 2015;48(2):403–410. doi: 10.3233/JAD-150437.

Chapter 6   Minerals and Toxicity: Lithium in Context
No references

Chapter 7   The History of Lithium in Medical Treatment

1. Strobusch AD, Jefferson JW. The checkered history of lithium in medicine. *Pharm Hist.* 1980;22(2):72–76.

2. Shorter E. The history of lithium therapy. *Bipolar Disord.* 2009;Suppl 2:4–9. doi: 10.1111/j.1399-5618.2009.00706.x.

3. Lange C. Bidrag til Urinsyrediatesens Klinik. *Hospitalstidende.* 1886;5:1–15, 21–38, 45–63, 69–83.

4. Cade JFJ. Lithium salts in the treatment of psychotic excitement. *Med J Aust.* 1949;36:349–352.

5. Schou M, Juel-Nielsen N, Strömgren E, Voldby H. The treatment of manic psychoses by the administration of lithium salts. *J Neurol Neurosurg Psychiatry.* 1954;17(4):250–60.

Chapter 8   The Cinderella Drug: Why We're Slow to Recognize Lithium's Value

1. Fels A. Should we all take a bit of lithium? *The New York Times.* www.nytimes.com/2014/09/14/opinion/sunday/

should-we-all-take-a-bit-of-lithium.html. September 13, 2014. Accessed August 12, 2018.

2. Goodwin JS, Goodwin JM. The tomato effect. Rejection of highly efficacious therapies. *JAMA*. 1984;251(18):2387–2390.

3. Macdonald A, Briggs K, Poppe M, et al. A feasibility and tolerability study of lithium in Alzheimer's disease. *Intl J Geriatr Psychiatry*. 2008; 23(7):704–711. doi: 10.1002/gps.1964.

4. Hampel, H, Ewers M, Bürger K, et al. Lithium trial in Alzheimer's disease: a randomized, single-blind, placebo-controlled, multicenter 10-week study. *J Clin Psychiatry*. 2009;70(6):922–931.

5. Forlenza OV, Diniz BS, Radanovic M, et al. Disease-modifying properties of long-term lithium treatment for amnestic mild cognitive impairment: Randomised controlled trial. *Br J Psychiatry*. 2011;198(5):351–356. doi: 10.1192/bjp.bp.110.080044.

Chapter 9   How Lithium Protects Against Alzheimer's

1. Sassi RB, Nicoletti M, Brambilla P, et al. Increased gray matter volume in lithium-treated bipolar disorder patients. *Neurosci Lett*. 2002 Aug 30;329(2):243–245.

2. Bearden CE, Thompson PM, Dutton RA, et al. Three-dimensional mapping of hippocampal anatomy in unmedicated and lithium-treated patients with bipolar disorder. *Neuropsychopharmacology*. 2008;33(6):1229–1238. doi: 10.1038/sj.npp.1301507

3. Kempton MJ, Geddes JR, Ettinger U, Williams SC, Grasby PM. Meta-analysis, database, and meta-regression of 98 structural imaging studies in bipolar disorder. *Arch Gen Psychiatry*. 2008;65(9):1017–1032. doi: 10.1001/archpsyc.65.9.1017.

4. Leyhe T, Eschweiler GW, Stransky E, et al. Increase of BDNF serum concentration in lithium treated patients with early Alzheimer's disease. *J Alzheimers Dis*. 2009;16(3):649–656. doi: 10.3233/JAD-2009-1004.

5. Walz JC, Frey BN, Andreazza AC, et al. Effects of lithium and valproate on serum and hippocampal neurotrophin-3 levels in

an animal model of mania. *J Psychiatr Res. 2008;*42(5):416–421. doi: 10.1016/j.jpsychires.2007.03.005

6. Fukumoto T, Morinobu S, Okamoto Y, Kagaya A, Yamawaki S. Chronic lithium treatment increases the expression of brain-derived neurotrophic factor in the rat brain. *Psychopharmacology (Berl).* 2001158(1):100–106. doi: 10.1007/s002130100871

7. Moffett JR, Ross B, Arun P, Madhavarao CN, Namboodiri AM. N-Acetylaspartate in the CNS: From neurodiagnostics to neurobiology [published online ahead of print January 5 2007]. *Progr Neurobiology.* 2007;81(2):89–131.

8. Yildiz-Yesiloglu A, Ankerst DP. Neurochemical alterations of the brain in bipolar disorder and their implications for pathophysiology: A systematic review of the in vivo proton magnetic resonance spectroscopy findings [published online ahead of print May 4 2006]. *Progr Neuropsychopharmacol Biol Psychiatry.* 2006;30(6):969. doi: 10.1016/j.pnpbp.2006.03.012

9. Forester BP, Finn CT, Berlow YA, et al. Brain lithium, N-acetyl aspartate and myo-inositol levels in older adults with bipolar disorder treated with lithium: a lithium-7 and proton magnetic resonance spectroscopy study. *Bipolar Disord.* 2008;10(6):691–700. doi: 10.1111/j.1399-5618.2008.00627.x.

10. Jope RS, Roh M. Glycogen synthase kinase-3 (GSK3) in psychiatric diseases and therapeutic interventions. *Curr Drug Targets.* 2006;7(11):1421–1434.

11. Hooper C, Killick R, Lovestone S. The GSK3 hypothesis of Alzheimer's disease [published online ahead of print December 18 2007]. *J Neurochem.* 2008;104(6):1433–1439.

12. Wada A. Lithium and neuropsychiatric therapeutics: neuroplasticity via glycogen synthase kinase-3.BETA, BETA.-catenin, and neurotrophin cascades [published online ahead of print May 8 2009]. *J Pharmacol Sci.* 2009;110(1):14–28.

13. Engel T, Goñi-Oliver P, Lucas JJ, Avila J, Hernández F. Chronic lithium administration to FTDP-17 tau and GSK-3beta overexpressing mice prevents tau hyperphosphorylation and

neurofibrillary tangle formation, but pre-formed neurofibrillary tangles do not revert [published online ahead of print October 24 2006]. *J Neurochem.* 2006;99(6):1445–1455.

14. Castillo-Quan JI, Li L, Kinghorn KJ, et al. Lithium promotes longevity through GSK3/NRF2-dependent hormesis [published online ahead of print April 7 2016]. *Cell Rep.* 2016;15(3):638–650. doi: 10.1016/j.celrep.2016.03.041.

15. Cheung ZH, Ip NY. Autophagy deregulation in neurodegenerative diseases – recent advances and future perspectives [published online ahead of print June 17 2011]. *J Neurochem.* 2011;118(3):317–325. doi: 10.1111/j.1471-4159.2011.07314.x.

16. Harwood AJ. Lithium and bipolar mood disorder: The inositol-depletion hypothesis revisited. *Mol Psychiatry.* 2005;10(1):117–126. doi: 10.1038/sj.mp.4001618.

17. Sarkar S, Floto RA, Berger Z, et al. Lithium induces autophagy by inhibiting inositol monophosphatase. *J Cell Biol.* 2005 Sep 26;170(7):1101–1111. doi: 10.1083/jcb.200504035

18. Ravikumar B, Sarkar S, Davies J, et al. Regulation of mammalian autophagy in physiology and pathophysiology. *Physiol Rev.* 2010;90(4):1383–435. doi: 10.1152/physrev.00030.2009.

19. Shimohama S. Apoptosis in Alzheimer's disease-an update. *Apoptosis.* 2000;5(1):9–16.

20. Liechti FD, Stüdle N, Theurillat R, et al. The mood-stabilizer lithium prevents hippocampal apoptosis and improves spatial memory in experimental meningitis. *Plos ONE.* 2014;9(11):e113607. doi: 10.1371/journal.pone.0113607. eCollection 2014.

21. Manji HK, Moore GJ, Chen G. Review: Lithium at 50: have the neuroprotective effects of this unique cation been overlooked? *Biol Psychiatry.* 1999;46(7):929–940.

22. Chen G, Zeng WZ, Yuan PX, et al. The mood-stabilizing agents lithium and valproate robustly increase the levels of the neuroprotective protein bcl-2 in the CNS. *J Neurochem.* 1999;72(2):879–882.

23. Hamilton A, Zamponi GW, Ferguson SG. Glutamate receptors function as scaffolds for the regulation of β-amyloid and cellular prion protein signaling complexes. *Mol Brain*. 2015;8:18. doi: 10.1186/s13041-015-0107-0.

24. Hashimoto R, Takei N, Shimazu K, et al. Lithium induces brain-derived neurotrophic factor and activates TrkB in rodent cortical neurons: An essential step for neuroprotection against glutamate excitotoxicity. *Neuropharmacology*. 2002;43(7):1173–1179.

25. Moore AH, O'Banion M. Neuroinflammation and anti-inflammatory therapy for Alzheimer's disease. *Adv Drug Deliv Rev*. 2002;54(12):1627–1656.

26. Nahman S, Belmaker R, Azab A. Effects of lithium on lipopolysaccharide-induced inflammation in rat primary glia cells [published online ahead of print October 12 2011]. *Innate Immun*. 2012;18(3):447–458. doi: 10.1177/1753425911421512.

27. Basselin M, Kim H-W, Chen M, et al. Lithium modifies brain arachidonic and docosahexaenoic metabolism in rat lipopolysaccharide model of neuroinflammation [published online ahead of print December 29 2009]. *J Lipid Res*. 2010;51(5):1049–1056. doi: 10.1194/jlr.M002469.

28. Wallace, J. Calcium dysregulation, and lithium treatment to forestall Alzheimer's disease - a merging of hypotheses [published online ahead of print February 22, 2014]. *Cell Calcium*. 2014;55(3):175–181. doi: 10.1016/j.ceca.2014.02.005.

29. Kubota T, Miyake K, Hirasawa T. Epigenetic understanding of gene-environment interactions in psychiatric disorders: a new concept of clinical genetics. *Clin Epigenetics*. 2012;4(1):1. doi: 10.1186/1868-7083-4-1.

30. Dwivedi T, Zhang H. Lithium-induced neuroprotection is associated with epigenetic modification of specific BDNF gene promoter and altered expression of apoptotic-regulatory proteins. *Front Neurosci*. 2015;8:457. doi: 10.3389/fnins.2014.00457.

31. Leyhe T, Eschweiler GW, Stransky E, et al. Increase of BDNF serum concentration in lithium treated patients with early

Alzheimer's disease. *J Alzheimers Dis.* 2009;16(3):649–656. doi: 10.3233/JAD-2009-1004.

32. Lee RS, Pirooznia M, Guintivano J, et al. Search for common targets of lithium and valproic acid identifies novel epigenetic effects of lithium on the rat leptin receptor gene. *Transl Psychiatry.* 2015;5:e600. doi: 10.1038/tp.2015.90.

33. Farah R, Khamisy-Farah R, Amit T, Youdim MB, Arraf Z. Lithium's gene expression profile, relevance to neuroprotection A cDNA microarray study [published online ahead of print January 17 2013]. *Cell Mol Neurobiol.* 2013;33(3):411–420. doi: 10.1007/s10571-013-9907-x.

Chapter 10   Lithium's Broader Benefits for Lifelong Brain Health

1. Chenu F, Bourin M. Potentiation of antidepressant-like activity with lithium: Mechanism involved. *Curr Drug Targets.* 2006;7(2):159–163.

2. Bschor T, Adli M, Baethge C, et al. Lithium augmentation increases the ACTH and cortisol response in the combined DEX/CRH test in unipolar major depression. *Neuropsychopharmacology.* 2002;27(3):470–478. doi: 10.1016/S0893-133X(02)00323-8.

3. Bschor T, Baethge C, Adli M, et al. Association between response to lithium augmentation and the combined DEX/CRH test in major depressive disorder. *J Psychiatric Res.* 2003;37(2):135–143.

4. Wegener G, Bandpey Z, Heiberg IL, Mørk A, Rosenberg R. Increased extracellular serotonin level in rat hippocampus induced by chronic citalopram is augmented by subchronic lithium: neurochemical and behavioural studies in the rat [published online ahead of print January 28 2003]. *Psychopharmacology (Berl).* 2003;166(2):188–194. doi: 0.1007/s00213-002-1341-6.

5. Price LH, Charney DS, Delgado PL, Heninger GR. Lithium and serotonin function: Implications for the serotonin hypothesis of depression. *Psychopharmacology (Berl).* 1990;100(1):3–12.

6. Beaulieu JM, Sotnikova TD, Yao WD, et al. Lithium antagonizes dopamine-dependent behaviors mediated by an AKT/glycogen

synthase kinase cascade [published online ahead of print March 24 2004]. *Proc Natl Acad Sci USA.* 2004;101(14):4099–4104. doi: 10.1073/pnas.0307921101.

7. Del' Guidice T, Beaulieu J. Selective disruption of dopamine D2-receptors/beta-arrestin2 signaling by mood stabilizers [published online ahead of print October 12 2015]. *J Recept Signal Transduct Res.* 2015;35(3):224–232. doi: 10.3109/10799893.2015.1072976.

8. Alia-Klein N, Goldstein RZ, Kriplani A, et al. Brain monoamine oxidase A activity predicts trait aggression. *J Neurosci.* 2008;28(19):5099–5104. doi: 10.1523/JNEUROSCI.0925-08.2008.

9. Fisar Z, Hroudova J, Raboch J. Inhibition of monoamine oxidase activity by antidepressants and mood stabilizers. *Neuro Endocrinol Lett.* 2010;31(5):645–656.

10. Mischley L. The role of lithium in neurological health and disease. *J Orthomol Med.* 2014;29(3):101.

11. Andreazza AC, Anna MK, Frey BN, et al. Oxidative stress markers in bipolar disorder: A meta-analysis [published online ahead of print June 9, 2008]. *J Affect Disord.* 2008;111(2–3):135–144. doi: 10.1016/j.jad.2008.04.013.

12. Cui J, Shao L, Young L, Wang J. Role of glutathione in neuroprotective effects of mood stabilizing drugs lithium and valproate [published online ahead of print December 19 2006]. *Neuroscience.* 2007;144(4):1447–1453. doi: 10.1016/j.neuroscience.2006.11.010.

13. DiMauro S, Davidzon G. Mitochondrial DNA and disease. *Ann Med.* 2005;33(3):222–232. doi: 10.1080/07853890510007368.

14. Struewing IT, Barnett CD, Tang T, Mao CD. Lithium increases PGC-1a expression and mitochondrial biogenesis in primary bovine aortic endothelial cells [published online ahead of print April 20 2007]. *FEBS J.* 2007;274(11):2749–2765. doi: 10.1111/j.1742-4658.2007.05809.x.

15. Forester BP, Finn CT, Berlow YA, et al. Brain lithium, N-acetyl aspartate and myo-inositol levels in older adults with bipolar

disorder treated with lithium: a lithium-7 and proton magnetic resonance spectroscopy study. *Bipolar Disord.* 2008;10(6):691–700. doi: 10.1111/j.1399-5618.2008.00627.x.

Chapter 11   The Fascinating History of Element 3: Water and Technology

1. El-Mallakh, RS, Roberts RJ. Lithiated lemon-lime sodas. *Am J Psychiatry.* 2007;164(11):1662. doi: 10.1176/appi.ajp.2007.07081255.

2. Georgotas A, Gershon S. Historical perspectives and current highlights on lithium treatment in manic-depressive illness. *J Clin Psychopharmacol.* 1981;1(1):27–31.

3. Schrauzer GN. Lithium: Occurrence, dietary intakes, nutritional essentiality. *J Am Coll Nutr.* 2002;21(1):14–21.

4. Schrauzer GN, Shrestha KP. Lithium in drinking water and the incidences of crimes, suicides, and arrests related to drug addictions. *Biol. Trace Elem. Res.* 1990;25:105–113. doi: 10.1007/BF02990271.

5. Ohgami H, Terao T, Shiotsuki I, Ishii N, Iwata N. Lithium levels in drinking water and risk of suicide. *Br J Psychiatry.* 2009;194:464–465. doi: 10.1192/bjp.bp.108.055798.

6. Sugawara N, Yasui-Furukori N, Ishii N, Iwata N, Terao T. Lithium in tap water and suicide mortality in Japan. *Int J Environ Res Public Health.* 2013;10(11):6044–6048. doi: 10.3390/ijerph10116044.

7. Jaskula BW. *U.S. Geological Survey, mineral commodity summaries-lithium.* Minerals.usgs.gov. https://minerals.usgs.gov/minerals/pubs/commodity/lithium/mcs-2015-lithi.pdf. January 2015. Accessed August 12, 2018.

8. O'Bannon, LS. *Dictionary of Ceramic Science and Engineering.* New York: Plenum Press; 1984.

9. Ratnakumar BV, Smart MC, Ewell RC, et al. Lithium-sulfur dioxide batteries on Mars rovers. Paper presented at: 2nd International Energy Conversion Engineering Conference, Providence, Rhode Island, August 15–18, 2004; Pasadena, CA: Jet Propulsion Laboratory, National Aeronautics and Space

Administration. https://trs.jpl.nasa.gov/handle/2014/38846. Accessed August 12, 2018.

Chapter 12   How to Make Lithium Part of Your Diet

1. Kling MA, Manowitz P, Pollack IW. Rat brain and serum lithium concentrations after acute injections of lithium carbonate and orotate. *J Pharm Pharmacol.* 1978 30(6):368–370.
2. Schrauzer GN. Lithium: Occurrence, dietary intakes, nutritional essentiality. *J Am Coll Nutr.* 2002;21(1):14–21.
3. Kronemann H, Anke M, Groppel B, Riedel E. The capacity of organs to indicate the lithium level. In: Anke M, Baumann W, Braünlich H, Brückner C (eds): Proceedings 4. Spurenelement Symposium 1983, Jena: VEB Kongressdruck, pp 85–93.
4. Watts DL. Nutrient interrelationships: minerals, vitamins, endocrines. *J Orthomol Med.* 1990;5(1):11–19.
5. Adams JB, Holloway CE, George F, Quig D. Analyses of toxic metals and essential minerals in the hair of Arizona children with autism and associated conditions, and their mothers. *Biol Trace Elem Res.* 2006;110(3):193–209. doi: 10.1385/BTER:110:3:193.

Chapter 13   The Dangers of Homocysteine and How to Measure It

1. Seshadri S, Beiser A, Selhub J, et al. Plasma homocysteine as a risk factor for dementia and Alzheimer's disease. *N Engl J Med.* 2002; 346(7):476–483. doi: 0.1056/NEJMoa011613.
2. Dawber, TR, Meadors GF, Moore FE Jr. Epidemiological approaches to heart disease: The Framingham Study. *Am J Public Health Nations Health.* 1951;41:279–281.
3. Ford AH, Flicker L, Alfonso H, et al. Plasma homocysteine and MTHFRC677T polymorphism as risk factors for incident dementia [published online ahead of print July 11 2011]. *J Neurol Neurosurg Psychiatry.* 2012;83(1):70–75. doi: 10.1136/jnnp.2011.242446.
4. Zylberstein DE, Lissner L, Björkelu C, et al. Midlife homocysteine and late-life dementia in women. A prospective population study

[published online ahead of print April 1 2009]. *Neurobiol Aging.* 2011;32(3):380–386. doi: 10.1016/j.neurobiolaging.2009.02.024.

5. Bengtsson C, Blohme G, Hallberg L, et al. The study of women in Gothenburg 1968-1969-a population study. General design, purpose and sampling results. *Acta Med Scand.* 1973;193:311–318.

6. Selhub J. The many facets of hyperhomocysteinemia: Studies from the Framingham cohorts. *J Nutr.* 2006;136(6 Suppl):1726S–1730S. doi: 10.1093/jn/136.6.1726S.

Chapter 14   Folic Acid and Other B Vitamins Lower Homocysteines

1. Homocysteine Lowering Trialists' Collaboration. Lowering blood homocysteine with folic acid based supplements: Meta-analysis of randomised trials. *BMJ.* 1998;316(7135):894–898.

Chapter 15   Vitamin D and Alzheimer's

1. Jayedi A, Rashidy-Pour A, Shab-Bidar S. Vitamin D status and risk of dementia and Alzheimer's disease: A meta-analysis of dose-response [published online ahead of print February 15 2018]. *Nutr Neurosci.* 2018;1–10. doi:10.1080/1028415x.2018.1436639.

2. Berridge MJ. Vitamin D deficiency accelerates ageing and age-related diseases: A novel hypothesis. *J Physiol.* 2017;595(22):6825–6836. doi:10.1113/jp274887.

3. Gezen-Ak D, Yilmazer S, Dursun E. The vitamin D in Alzheimer's disease? The hypothesis. *J Alzheimers Dis.* 2014;40:257–269. doi: 10.3233/JAD-131970.

4. Annweiler C, Rolland Y, Schott AM, et al. Higher vitamin D dietary intake is associated with lower risk of Alzheimer's disease: A 7-year follow up. *J Gerontol A Bi Sci Med Sci.* 2012;67(11):1205–1211. doi: 10.1093/gerona/gls107.

5. Littlejohns TJ, Henley WE, Lang IA, et al. Vitamin D and the risk of dementia and Alzheimer's disease. *Neurology.* 2014;83(10):920–928. doi: 10.1212/WNL.0000000000000755.

Chapter 16   Curcumin: Anti-Inflammatory and Antioxidant

1. Vas CJ, Pinto C, Panikker D, et al. Prevalence of dementia in an urban Indian population. *Int Psychogeriatr.* 2001;13(4):439–450.

2. Hamaguchi T, Ono K, Yamada M. Curcumin and Alzheimer's disease. *CNS Neurosci Ther.* 2010;16(5):285–297. doi: 10.1111/j.1755-5949.2010.00147.x.

3. Small GW, Siddarth P, Li Z, et al. Memory and brain amyloid and tau effects of a bioavailable form of curcumin in non-demented adults: A double-blind, placebo-controlled 18-month trial [published online ahead of print October 27 2017]. *Am J Geriatr Psychiatry.* 2018;26(3):266–277. doi: 10.1016/j.jagp.2017.10.010.

4. Lopresti AL, Maes M, Maker GL, Hood SD, Drummond PD. Curcumin for the treatment of major depression: A randomised, double-blind, placebo controlled study [published online ahead of print June 11 2014]. *J Affect Disord.* 2014;167: 368–375. doi: 10.1016/j.jad.2014.06.001.

5. Lim GP, Chu T, Yang F, et al. The curry spice curcumin reduces oxidative damage and amyloid pathology in an Alzheimer transgenic mouse. *J Neurosci.* 2001;21(21):8370–8377.

6. Prasad S, Tyagi AK, Aggarwal BB. Recent Developments in delivery, bioavailability, absorption and metabolism of curcumin: the golden pigment from golden spice [published online ahead of print January 15, 2014]. *Cancer Res Treat.* 2014;46(1):2–18. doi: 10.4143/crt.2014.46.1.2.

Chapter 17   NAC Protects Along Multiple Pathways

1. Hara Y, McKeehan N, Dacks PA, Fillit HM. Evaluation of the neuroprotective potential of N-acetylcysteine for prevention and treatment of cognitive aging and dementia. *J Prev Alzheimers Dis.* 2017;4(3):201–206. doi: 10.14283/jpad.2017.22.

2. da Costa M, Bernardi J, Costa L, et al. N-acetylcysteine treatment attenuates the cognitive impairment and synaptic plasticity loss induced by streptozotocin [published online ahead

of print May 9 2017]. *Chem Biol Interact.* 2017;272:37–46. doi: 10.1016/j.cbi.2017.05.008.

3. Farr SA, Poon HF, Dogrukol-Ak D, et al. The antioxidants alpha-lipoic acid and N-acetylcysteine reverse memory impairment and brain oxidative stress in aged SAMP8 mice. *J Neurochem.* 2003;84(5):1173–1183.

4. Remington R, Lortie JJ, Hoffmann H, et al. A nutritional formulation for cognitive performance in mild cognitive impairment: A placebo-controlled trial with an open-label extension. *J Alzheimers Dis.* 2015;48(3):591–595. doi: 10.3233/JAD-150057.

5. Chan A, Remington R, Kotyla E, et al. A vitamin/nutriceutical formulation improves memory and cognitive performance in community-dwelling adults without dementia. *J Nutr Health Aging.* 2010;14(3):224–230.

6. Adair JC, Knoefel JE, Morgan N. Controlled trial of N-acetylcysteine for patients with probable Alzheimer's disease. *Neurology.* 2001;57(8):1515–1517.

7. Skvarc DR, Dean OM, Byrne LK, et al. The effect of N-acetylcysteine (NAC) on human cognition – A systematic review [published online ahead of print April 21 2017]. *Neurosci Biobehav Rev.* 2017;78:44–56. doi: 10.1016/j.neubiorev.2017.04.013.

8. McCaddon A, Hudson PR, Cummings JL. Exploring novel treatment options: Cognitive decline in Alzheimer's disease. *CNS Spectr.* 2010;15(1):1–7.

Chapter 18   Brain Foods: Blueberries, Grape Seed, and Green Tea

1. Krikorian R, Shidler M, Nash T, Kalt W, et al. Blueberry supplementation improves memory in older adults. *J Agric Food Chem.* 2010;58(7):3996–4000. doi: 10.1021/jf9029332.

2. Boespflug EL, Eliassen JC, Dudley JA, et al. Enhanced neural activation with blueberry supplementation in mild cognitive impairment [published online ahead of print

February 21 2017]. *Nutr Neurosci.* 2018;21(4):297–305. doi: 10.1080/1028415X.2017.1287833.

3. Miller MG, Hamilton DA, Joseph JA, Shukitt-Hale B. Dietary blueberry improves cognition among older adults in a randomized, double-blind, placebo-controlled trial [published online ahead of print March 10 2017]. *Eur J Nutr.* 2018;57(3):1169–1180. doi: 10.1007/s00394-017-1400-8.

4. Whyte A, Schafer G, Williams C. Cognitive effects following acute wild blueberry supplementation in 7- to 10-year-old children [published online ahead of print October 5 2015]. *Eur J Nutr.* 2016;55(6):2151–2162. doi: 10.1007/s00394-015-1029-4.

5. Schrager MA, Hilton J, Gould R, Kelly VE. Effects of blueberry supplementation on measures of functional mobility in older adults [published online ahead of print January 12 2015]. *Appl Physiol Nutr Metab.* 2015;40(6):543–549. doi: 10.1139/apnm-2014-0247.

6. Wang Y, Thomas P, Zhong J, et al. Consumption of grape seed extract prevents amyloid-beta deposition and attenuates inflammation in brain of an Alzheimer's disease mouse [published online ahead of print February 10 2009]. *Neurotox Res.* 2009;15(1):3–14. doi: 10.1007/s12640-009-9000-x.

7. Borgwardt S, Hammann F, Scheffler K, et al. Neural effects of green tea extract on dorsolateral prefrontal cortex [published online ahead of print August 29 2012]. *Eur J Clin Nutr.* 2012;66(11):1187–1192. doi: 10.1038/ejcn.2012.105.

8. Feng L, Chong MS, Lim WS, et al. Tea consumption reduces the incidence of neurocognitive disorders: Findings from the Singapore longitudinal aging study. *J Nutr Health Aging.* 2016;20(10):1002–1009. doi: 10.1007/s12603-016-0687-0.

9. Hyung S, DeToma AS, Brender JR, et al. Insights into antiamyloidogenic properties of the green tea extract (-)-epigallocatechin-3-gallate toward metal-associated amyloid-β species [published online ahead of print February 20 2013]. *Proc Natl Acad Sci USA.* 2013;110(10):3743–3748. doi: 10.1073/pnas.1220326110.

10. McCaddon A, Hudson PR, Cummings JL. Exploring novel treatment options: cognitive decline in Alzheimer's disease. *CNS Spectr.* 2010;15(1):1–7.

Chapter 19   A Golden Public Health Intervention

1. Phelps J. Lithium for Alzheimer prevention: What are we waiting for? *Psychiatric Times.* www.psychiatrictimes.com/psychopharmacology/lithium-alzheimer-prevention-what-are-we-waiting. October 7, 2016. Accessed August 12, 2018.

2. Schrauzer GN, Shrestha KP. Lithium in drinking water and the incidences of crimes, suicides, and arrests related to drug addictions. *Biol. Trace Elem Res.* 1990;25:105–113. doi: 10.1007/BF02990271.

3. Ohgami H, Terao T, Shiotsuki I, Ishii N, Iwata N. Lithium levels in drinking water and risk of suicide. *Br J Psychiatry.* 2009;194(5):464–465; discussion 446. doi: 10.1192/bjp.bp.108.055798.

4. Giotakos O, Nisianakis P, Tsouvelas G, Giakalou V. Lithium in the public water supply and suicide mortality in Greece [published online ahead of print September 27, 2013]. *Biol Trace Elem Res.* 2013;156(1-3):376–379. doi: 10.1007/s12011-013-9815-4.

5. Helbich M, Leitner M, Kapusta ND. Geospatial examination of lithium in drinking water and suicide mortality. *Int J Health Geogr.* 2012;11:19. doi: 10.1186/1476-072X-11-19

6. Lewitzka U, Severus E, Bauer R, et al. The suicide prevention effect of lithium: More than 20 years of evidence—a narrative review [published online ahead of print July 18 2015]. *Int J Bipolar Disord.* 2015;3(1):32. doi: 10.1186/s40345-015-0032-2.

7. Song J, Sjölander A, Joas E, et al. Suicidal behavior during lithium and valproate treatment: A within-individual 8-year prospective study of 50,000 patients with bipolar disorder [published online ahead of print June 9 2017]. *Am J Psychiatry.* 2017;174(8):795–802. doi:10.1176/appi.ajp.2017.16050542

8. Kessing LV, Gerds TA, Knudsen NN, et al. Association of lithium in drinking water with the incidence of dementia. *JAMA Psychiatry.* 2017;74(10):1005–1010. doi: 10.1001/jamapsychiatry.2017.2362.

9. McGrath JJ, Berk M. Could lithium in drinking water reduce the incidence of dementia? *JAMA Psychiatry.* 2017;74(10):983–984. doi: 10.1001/jamapsychiatry.2017.2336.

10. Fels A. Should we all take a bit of lithium? *The New York Times.* www.nytimes.com/2014/09/14/opinion/sunday/should-we-all-take-a-bit-of-lithium.html. September 13, 2014. Accessed August 12, 2018.

Chapter 20   Conclusion: Lithium and Happier Aging

1. Buettner D. *The Blue Zones: Lessons For Living Longer From the People Who've Lived The Longest.* Washington, D.C.: National Geographic Society; 2010.

PSYCHIATRY REDEFINED

BOOK SERIES

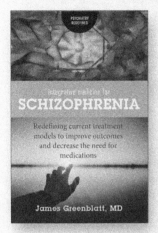

integrative medicine for
SCHIZOPHRENIA

Redefining current treatment
models to improve outcomes
and decrease the need for
medications

James Greenblatt, MD

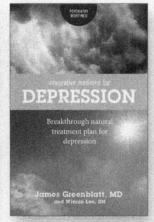

integrative medicine for
DEPRESSION

Breakthrough natural
treatment plan for
depression

James Greenblatt, MD
and Winnie Lee, RN

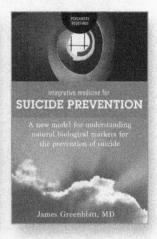

integrative medicine for
SUICIDE PREVENTION

A new model for understanding
natural biological markers for
the prevention of suicide

James Greenblatt, MD

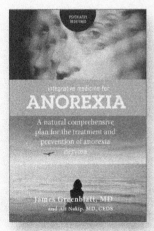

integrative medicine for
ANOREXIA

A natural comprehensive
plan for the treatment and
prevention of anorexia
nervosa

James Greenblatt, MD
and Ali Nakip, MD, CKDS

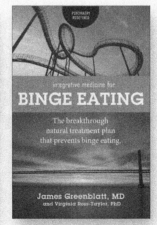

integrative medicine for
BINGE EATING

The breakthrough
natural treatment plan
that prevents binge eating.

James Greenblatt, MD
and Virginia Ross-Taylor, PhD

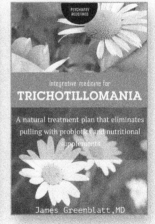

integrative medicine for
TRICHOTILLOMANIA

A natural treatment plan that eliminates
pulling with probiotics and nutritional
supplements

James Greenblatt, MD

ADDITIONAL

BOOKS BY

THE AUTHOR

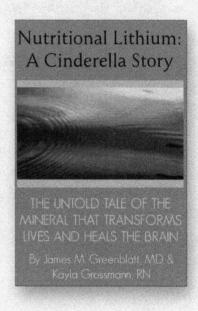

Nutritional Lithium:
A Cinderella Story

THE UNTOLD TALE OF THE
MINERAL THAT TRANSFORMS
LIVES AND HEALS THE BRAIN

By James M. Greenblatt, MD &
Kayla Grossmann, RN

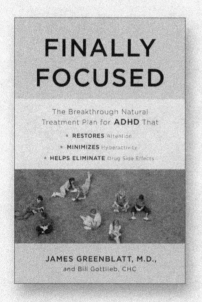

FINALLY
FOCUSED

The Breakthrough Natural
Treatment Plan for **ADHD** That

* **RESTORES** Attention
* **MINIMIZES** Hyperactivity
* **HELPS ELIMINATE** Drug Side Effects

JAMES GREENBLATT, M.D.,
and Bill Gottlieb, CHC

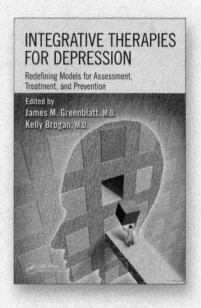

INTEGRATIVE THERAPIES
FOR DEPRESSION

Redefining Models for Assessment,
Treatment, and Prevention

Edited by
James M. Greenblatt, M.D.
Kelly Brogan, M.D.

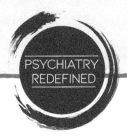

We Can Do Better

It is no secret that the current symptomatic treatment model of mental illness is not supporting our patients in recovery or wellness.

The field of psychiatry has lagged far behind in understanding the value of integrative medicine in the treatment of mental illness. This lag has created a wedge between patients and their healthcare providers.

Psychiatry Redefined acts as a bridge between patients and their healthcare providers, family members, and caregivers, that widens the possibilities of treating and sustaining mental health.

Psychiatry Redefined is a vision for mental health professionals, patients, family, and caregivers.

Psychiatry Redefined is dedicated to patients suffering from ineffective treatments, exhausted by their experience, and seeking more individualized care.

We Have To Do Better

James Greenblatt, MD

Please visit our website for more information

WWW.PSYCHIATRYREDEFINED.ORG

CPSIA information can be obtained
at www.ICGtesting.com
Printed in the USA
LVHW051832261119
638404LV00003B/72/P

9 781525 539985